M

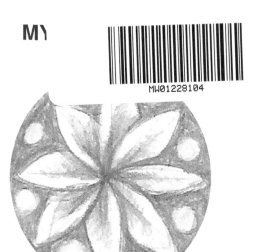

I love myself and the world loves me back.
I believe in myself and the world believes in me
back.
I heal myself and the world heals me back.
I am joyful so the world is joyful.
Because I know that we are one, I also know that
when I am love, you are love and we are love.
**I am effortless creation, and I create everything
that brings me joy.**

Introduction

The Path to Heal is a healing modality, which removes all blocks to choosing joy, leading to an abundance of health, wealth and happiness. Up until now, to receive help through the dimensions of **The Path to Heal**, one would need to visit a **Path** practitioner. Practitioners would walk the client through the dimensions using their guidance bringing the client to the understanding of blocks.

This book is set up so that you have the opportunity to discover your blocks to joy by yourself. By using these protocols, you trust your own guidance to lead you through a process similar to what a **Path** practitioner would do. As you proceed through these protocols, you release the shame and guilt that is obstructing your ability to choose happiness.

Trust what you discover while using this book. Trust your guidance. Trust the process. And at the end of it, your health conditions and unwanted circumstances can naturally release, as you actualize your true self, embracing what makes you happy.

*You have within you all the magic that you need to create a joyful, happy, healthy, prosperous life. This book and **The Path to Heal**, simply help you get out of your own way by clearing the unconscious blocks to happiness. The blocks evolve because our loved-ones and communities feel safe believing that life has to be hard to be worthwhile because love, optimism, hope and cheer feel too vulnerable. When the blocks are cleared, you upgrade your entire world using the currency of love, self-acceptance and joy and then all is always well. This evolution allows you to love yourself unconditionally and therefore compassion replaces judgment. Then you know that when I love you, you love me back.*

This book was developed with the help of Lisa Orlandi, a very gifted student and friend. Lisa helped me develop and trial each protocol. She filled the process of creating this book with joy.

Instructions

- The protocols within are self-help tools that helps you understand your blocks to joy. Once understood, the blocks release.
- You use guidance to make choices in this book.
- To use your guidance, you may:
  - Sniff lemon essential oil or hold clear quartz to help you receive clear guidance
  - Breathe in and trust the first answer that comes to mind
  - Dowse by using a pendulum or muscle testing (instructions on dowsing found later in this book)
- In this book, you use guidance to:
  - Choose a self-help protocol listed on the Table of Contents to help you release an issue. (Or randomly flip to a page)
  - Make choices within a protocol. Choices come in the form of:
    - words separated by "/" within parentheses – *choose one or more words*
    - words following diamond shaped bullet points – *choose one or more bullets*
    - fill in the blank over an underscored word – *fill in the blank with the first word that comes to mind*
- The understanding of the protocols will always come to you. You are being spiritually guided through this process. Internal shifts occur when the insight is received and then external doors open to facilitate your path to joy. When this shift occurs, you will have complete love and compassion for those still in pain and your love will guide them to their path to joy.

Tools

There are four tools that are recommended for use with these protocols: wild orange essential oil, lemon essential oil, quartz crystal and the 432 Hz Tuning Fork. These tools connect us to our essence which is love, thereby strengthening confidence. Additionally, these tools balance our hormonal function so that our body supports our joyful path.

- Wild orange and lemon essential oils are recommended in some of these protocols. Sniffing oils will expedite the healing by raising your vibration to unconditional love.
  - wild orange makes it easy for us to give love to others and makes it also easy for others to love you back – wild orange is the medicine that we need to believe that bliss is truly bliss
  - lemon helps us recognize the awesomeness of the vibration of love and therefore replaces fear with love in us an around us
- Quartz amplifies
  - self as the Divine Creator powered by self-love
  - the transmutation of karma to compassion
  - the love that is always available
  - joyful ownership of our divine gifts
- The Serenity 432 Hz tuning fork creates mathematic consistency with Heaven on Earth amplifying:
  - seamless manifestation from the heart, aligning your energy to bliss
  - alignment with the divine self so that you trust choices made from love rather than fear
  - self-acceptance
  - the recoding of our genes to release the genetic predisposition for pain, stress and struggle
- To work with the tuner and the quartz, you will be asked to perform the following motions with the healing tool in hand. *The symbol awakens our soul code so that we remember the "I Am". I Am divine. I Am all that is. I Am the grace of god. And most importantly, I Am love.*

  - Activate the tuning fork or hold the quartz, then quickly do the following movements:
  - 3 quick circles over right eye
  - Draw a sidesways "s" to get to the left eye
  - 3 quick circles over left eye
  - It is easy to purchase a 432 Hz tuning fork on-line. *It is not referred to elsewhere with the name Serenity.*

You can also find a recording of this tuning fork on www.thepathtoheal.com/sound and then click on link to access recordings.

Teaching Yourself To Dowse

Dowsing is a process of asking yes/no questions to your heart and higher self to receive the answer that helps you heal.

Go to www.thepathtoheal.com, books tab, scroll down to the bottom to view a muscle testing video demonstration.

Muscle testing: the easiest form of dowsing

- Make a ring on each hand with your thumb and index finger. Then link these two rings together.
- Create a little tension between the two rings. Set the intention that you will receive a "yes" answer when your hands separate with ease, and a "no" answer when you feel some tension between your two hands.
- Ask a simple yes/no question that you know the answer to, such as: "Is my name Rebecca"?
- After asking, pull your fingers apart and see if your hands separate with ease, or whether you feel tension and your hands remain linked.
- Ask multiple yes/no questions until you can feel the difference between a yes and a no.
- When muscle testing, there are absolute rules for success:
  a. Always go with your first "yes"; don't double check. If you double check, you'll likely get a different answer, as you've created doubt.
  b. The first yes is always correct.
  c. If muscle testing doesn't come easily, fake it until you make it: you're faking it is your inner voice giving you the right answers anyway!

There are many forms of muscle testing not described here. Feel free to use any method that works for you.

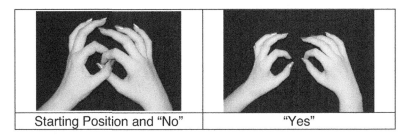

| Starting Position and "No" | "Yes" |

Pendulum:

- You can use any pendulum that you own or decide to purchase.
- Set the intention that the pendulum swings clockwise for a yes, and counterclockwise for a no.
- Ask questions as suggested above to practice using your pendulum.
- If you already communicate with your pendulum in a different manner, or if your pendulum wants to give you yes/no in a different manner, allow the energies to teach you how to use your pendulum.

Freedom (Healing Fear)

Fear is released when we have complete compassion for self because then there is nothing to be afraid of. Compassion allows us to be enthusiastically be ourselves, and then we are free to live the life of our dreams.

1) *Identity fears from list below then*
   Serenity Tuning Fork

2) *Dowse protocols in this book to help gain compassion for self thus allowing yourself to live in truth, which yields fearless freedom.*
3) *This results in the seamless manifestation of a peaceful and spectacular life.*

Are you afraid of:	√
not having enough money / disappointing someone	
change / surprises / unpredictability / technology	
being at fault / unfair blame / persecuted / getting fired	
Intimacy / sexuality / other's needs / not belonging	
social situations / gossip / viciousness / not being loved	
being followed / stalked / attacked / intruders	
being late / too much going on / out of control / being out of my routine	
breaking the rules and then looking like a fool / rejection	
confrontation / criticism / not getting approval / being manipulated	
disappointment / bumps / emptiness / crowded spaces / driving	
expressing my tastes and desires / my appetites / boredom	
heights / falling / addiction / getting hurt / driving	
letting my guard down / pleasure / relaxation	
no end in sight / never getting better / not having a meaningful life	
not getting enough sleep / lack of energy / not being able to breathe	
public speaking / popularity / not having down time	
not being up to the task / spatial challenges / being confused	
tragedy / accidents / someone else dying / disasters	
abandonment / loss / loss of power / losing / not being successful	
accountability / responsibility / success / being forgotten / not making a mark	
bad news / other's energy / never being well / my mental health	
being judged / being exposed / being smeared / the angry mob	
being too busy / not getting to relax / throwing things away	
being uncomfortable / not getting my needs met / pain	
not solving the problem (my problems or others')	
creepy crawlers / being overly influenced / being too indulgent	
dying / the dark / not being able to breathe / being stuck in the muck	
flying / flying away / not being good enough / imperfections	
getting old / illness / getting sick / body not working	
losing what I have / being replaced / other's motives	
making decisions / taking risks / making mistakes / something going wrong	
my own behavior / sinning / quiet / being still / thoughts	
not being heard / misinformation	
not pleasing others / body imperfections / being humiliated	
dogs or other animals	
spending money / having money / debt	
the unrecognizable / peacefulness / not being happy	

Self-help Protocols

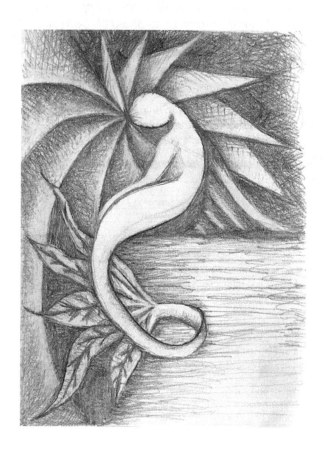

A Lovely Existence

1) I deny myself: *(dowse one or more below)*
    1. fitness and a comfortable body weight because I think it will make others jealous
    2. affluence because I think it will make me greedy
    3. appreciation because I think it will make me feel ungenerous
    4. attractiveness because I think it will make me inaccessible
    5. authenticity because I don't think I'm enough
    6. comfort because I think it will get me in trouble for not being tough
    7. confidence because I hate to visibly fail
    8. ease because I think it will make me soft
    9. easy manifestation because I think it will make life too unmotivating
    10. food because I think it will make me fat
    11. freedom because I think that a lack of rules creates chaos
    12. friends because I think it will make me scattered
    13. fun because I think it will make me disrespectful
    14. genius because I think it will separate me
    15. greatness because I think it will make me arrogant
    16. happiness because I think it will make time pass too fast
    17. health and a pain-free existence because I think it will make me unempathetic and unrelatable
    18. joy because I think it will make me lazy
    19. love because I think it will make me vulnerable
    20. money because I think it will make me self-centered
    21. my memory because I think it will make me sad and angry
    22. peace because others may find me dumb and naïve
    23. productivity because I think it will make me too in demand
    24. rejoicing because others are still sad
    25. romance because I would be devastated if I lost it
    26. self-respect because I think it will make me pushy
    27. self-worth because then I would have to breaks ties with loved ones who don't value me
    28. sexuality because I think it will make me a cheater
    29. sovereignty (free-choice) because my mistakes might be my fault (no one to blame)
    30. spirited movement because I might abandon my loved-ones
    31. strength because I think it will make me too independent
    32. trust because I think I will stop trying
    33. understanding because I'm too afraid of we'll discover inside of us
    34. visibility because I think it will create expectations
    35. vitality because then I won't have time for you

    therefore I am denying pleasurable success because I think it will bury me inside of exhaustive expectations leading to stress, anxiety and depression.

2) What if relaxing into complete generosity to self, leading to pleasurable success, never yields the sins or fears of the ego, because abundance created from the heart yields only love? Instead, I energize the shift into abundant pleasure knowing that it is within pleasure that we create an authentically loving and lovely existence.

Aligning my Ego to my Heart

Quartz crystal

1) My heart wants wondrous things. When my ego and heart align, then my desires manifest with synchronistic ease.

2) My heart wants first thought that come to mind.

3) My ego's fear gets in the way of my heart's desires because I'm afraid to fully actualize what's in my heart, because loved-ones did not want this for me. My authentic desires diverge from what loved-one(s) wanted for me because my loved-one's ego projects their unfulfilled desires and fears onto me.

4) Going against expectations scare me because I don't want to be rejected and alone. Thus, I have unconsciously created blocks to manifestation, actualizing as:
   ❖ viruses / health crises / exhaustion
   ❖ joint pain / body pain / headaches / cough
   ❖ lack of money / lack of success / feeling left out
   ❖ depression / unhappiness / anxiety / low self-esteem
   ❖ gastro-intestinal issues / organ trauma
   ❖ isolation / lack of intimacy / entitlement / complaints
   ❖ soul contracts that aren't serving me
   ❖ unbreakable habits / phobias / inflexibility
   ❖ emotion dysregulation / procrastination

5) What if I'm able to release my ego's fear of rejection because I can now recognize that my heart is true? When I allow myself to align with my heart, I am rewarded with joyful creations that are good for all.

6) As I create what's good for all, the universe surrounds me with authentic partners that embrace all that I am and all that I can be. I'm now ready to actualize my heart's wondrous desires because the world is waiting for me to lead by embracing joyful authenticity.

Serenity Tuning Fork

All That is Good

Quartz crystal ☺/☺

1) I have not let my spirit be joyously all that it can be, because then I would have to jump into fearlessness, trusting my heart, rather than my petrified mind.

2) When I reframe my existence to helping myself and others achieve their best lives, using my naturally gifted qualities, I fear that this change may be judged as inappropriate by traditional norms. Therefore, my ego wants to do the traditional thing so I don't get rejected. Moral judgment (which is often about fear) is not always loving. However, because I fear moral judgment from loved-one, I block self-actualization, leading to stagnation, in an attempt to fit in.

3) Stagnation creates spiritual blocks, thus blocking the manifestation of:
   ❖ good health
   ❖ loving relationships
   ❖ life affirming work
   ❖ financial freedom
   ❖ popularity
   ❖ self-confidence
   ❖ my gifts and value
   ❖ kindness and warmth
   ❖ a healed world

4) What if I give myself the courage to embrace my authentic vocation, knowing that I am a divine blessing which leads to my happiness, other's happiness and the manifestation of all that is good? And so I do.

Serenity Tuning Fork

An Extraordinary Life

1) I want to be successful and happily thriving but I hit roadblocks and can't fully manifest:
   ❖ good health
   ❖ loving relationships / easy relationships
   ❖ life affirming work
   ❖ financial freedom
   This lack of empowerment is driven by blocks to (drive/confidence/ease/resiliency/flexibility/curiosity/ passion/energy/optimism/self-respect).

2) My blocks formed because I wasn't given encouragement for my authentic (drive/confidence/ease/resiliency/flexibility/ curiosity/ passion/energy/optimism) by loved-one.

3) This lack of encouragement caused me to shut-down because strongly displaying my authentic empowerment causes me to feel like I might get abandoned for my individual strengths. I have now embraced my loved-ones values as my own to avoid feeling my wounded pain. This inauthenticity has developed into an allergy to:
   ❖ foods / dairy / gluten
   ❖ caffeine / drugs / alcohol
   ❖ pollen / grass / trees / smoke / chemicals
   ❖ animals / infectious allergens

4) What if it's just wrong when it comes to choosing loved-one's values over my values because it leads to a lack of flow blocking health and happiness? What if I allow me to love all of me, all of the time which leads to health, wealth and happiness? And what if I have just discovered the key to an extraordinary life?

Quartz crystal ☺/☺

And So I Do

1) I hold myself back with
   - ❖ bad moods / feeling like a victim
   - ❖ setting the bar too high or too low
   - ❖ joint pain / illness / allergies / sensitivities / headaches
   - ❖ everything hurts / teeth pain
   - ❖ insecurity / sensory issues / lack of connection / isolation
   - ❖ avoidance / memory issues
   - ❖ anxiety / panic / depression / neck pain
   - ❖ relationship issues
   - ❖ mobility issues / weight issues
   - ❖ schedule changes / cancellations / break-downs
   - ❖ irrational thought complexes
   - ❖ money issues / unenjoyable work
   - ❖ feeling like I'm broken
   - ❖ constant problems / focusing on world-wide problems
   - ❖ lack / lack of comfort / lack of time / lack of energy
   - ❖ (identity/personal/communal/world) crisis

   because I believe that my bold expression conflicts with my (self/family/community/work)'s unconscious need for misery and struggle so that:
   - ❖ prayer is necessary
   - ❖ there is a savior
   - ❖ we stay bonded through trauma, fear and betrayal
   - ❖ problem solving gives us meaning
   - ❖ we become political to "solve" our problems which allow us to bond in a common ideology
   - ❖ I remain relevant
   - ❖ I have to strategize in order to co-exist and survive (which makes me feel strong and wise)

2) However, this act of holding back is a lack of self-love, and is actualizing as lack. What if I transcend fear and allow myself to remember that embodying my bold and shiny gifts always creates connection, joy, fulfillment and abundance for my loved ones, my communities and the world? And so I do.

Quartz crystal ☉☉

Attentive Joy

Quartz crystal ⊘⊘

1) I'm annoyed by loved-one for being:
    ❖ tone deaf / not listening / a bully
    ❖ too loud and taking up too much space
    ❖ cranky / distrustful / conspiratorial / mean
    ❖ clueless / a tool / too devoted
    ❖ intrusive / persistent / unhelpful / too demanding
    ❖ distant / incomplete / without an answer
    ❖ talkative / passionate / sexual
    ❖ self-absorbed / an advantage taker/ a player
    ❖ needy / particular / a blamer / irrational
    ❖ manipulative / promoting fear
    ❖ deflective of responsibility / indecisive
    ❖ chaotic / too busy / unenergetic / flakey
    ❖ cocky / superior / disrespectful
    ❖ unaware of my feelings / unresponsive / inconsistent / flakey
    ❖ capricious / unreliable
    ❖ stuck in the same story (as the victim)
    ❖ uncaring / unforgiving / punishing
    ❖ pushy / in charge / irresistible
    ❖ imperfect / uncooperative
    ❖ inauthentic / untruthful / unclear / unavailable / critical
    ❖ lazy / pathetic / worn out / visibly pained / slow

2) In fact, because everything is a mirror of me, my annoyance simply exists because I yearn for my loved-one to fully share attentive joy and respect with me.

3) Once I recognize what I'm yearning for, my pain begins to heal. It is at this moment that I choose to give myself attentive joy and kindness by being emotionally connected and aware of my own needs. My awareness:
    • allows the recognition of my intrinsic value
    • allows the universe to align with the vibration of my heart and then my needs are easily fulfilled in lovingly magnificent ways
I now have room for others and my relationships become respectful and attentive joy.

Audaciously Bold

Sniff wild orange

1) There is a piece of me that is afraid to be boldly me because I may experience soul crushing rejection from first thought that comes to mind. Instead of being bold, my inner bully hides part of my identity.

2) In truth, it's easier to be authentically bold then in hiding. In order to hide my identity, I energetically restrain my bold expression with:
   ❖ sickness / body pain / headaches
   ❖ addiction / weight
   ❖ lack of money / losing my job
   ❖ lack of success / downturns
   ❖ feeling misunderstood and lonely
   ❖ hyperactivity / angst / micromanagement / obsession
   ❖ worries / fear
   ❖ waiting
   ❖ fighting / bitter stories / conflict / wars / revenge
   ❖ bad memories
   ❖ stressful situations / out of control situations
   ❖ being unrelaxed / lack of sleep
   ❖ being overly humble
   ❖ other's: pushiness / punishment

3) However, the sacred truth is that joy comes from being audaciously true to self, because love is always stronger than judgment and hate. Self-love (which is the absence of fear) always wins over the inner bully, because the inner bully is fueled by fear.

4) When I exist as self-love, communities rise up to support my love-being, because love begets love. And the more audaciously bold I get, then I create community by supporting others to boldly own their true identities. Now we are authentically healthy, peaceful, connected, abundant, successful, fulfilled and happy-go-lucky.

Quartz crystal

Breaking the Cycle

Serenity Tuning Fork

1) Because _{loved-one} wasn't proud of and dismissive of my:
   - ❖ special qualities
   - ❖ intelligence / intellectualism
   - ❖ work ethic / productiveness
   - ❖ kindness
   - ❖ accomplishments / success / skill/ gifts
   - ❖ company / fun
   - ❖ love / romance
   - ❖ point of view / choices / interests / voice
   - ❖ presence
   - ❖ personality
   - ❖ sexuality
   - ❖ spirituality

   my severely wounded self-esteem "asks" the ego to take over to limit criticism by:
   - ❖ retelling myself the bitter stories starring me as the victim and you as just wrong
   - ❖ perfectionism / analysis paralysis/overwork
   - ❖ leaning into insecurity
   - ❖ competing to be the best
   - ❖ isolating myself / depression
   - ❖ disassociation
   - ❖ shutting myself down with: sickness/body pain/allergies/fatigue
   - ❖ lying / hyperbole
   - ❖ putting myself down / perfectionism
   - ❖ focusing on other's flaws to create a sense of betterment for me
   - ❖ procrastination / lack of motivation
   - ❖ sickness / body pain
   - ❖ numbing my wounded pride with addictions

2) The solution is to give myself a break and continually see the best in me every day. As I do this, my self-pride increases. Then it's natural for me to show pride to others (because the competition to be the best is gone). I have broken the cycle.

3) I am the creator of a healed world.

Sniff wild orange

Bright Shiny Light of Love

Serenity Tuning Fork

1) My heart is afraid because I fear that I will lose _{first thought that} _{comes to mind}.. But what I'm really afraid of is losing is the (joy/love/grace/stillness/peace/fun) that I receive from you. This fear is lodged in my:
   - ❖ lungs/heart/liver/spleen/intestines/bladder/kidney
   - ❖ skin/hair/nails
   - ❖ system: digestive/cardiovascular/cerebrospinal/ endocrine/immune/lymphatic/muscular/nervous/ reproductive/skeletal/urinary
   and is making me uncomfortable and sick.

2) What if I remember that joy, love, grace, stillness, peace and fun are always available to me in an abundant and healthy way, because I can give this to me? And when I do, I have opened a door for others to share joy, love, grace, stillness, peace and fun because it's easy and it feels just right.

3) I am ready to release my fear of loss because I can never lose joy, love, grace, stillness, peace and fun, because I am a bright shiny light of love.

Quartz crystal

Center of Truth

1) Trauma gets stuck inside of us when we believe that we are somehow responsible for the traumatizing event.

2) Even though I know that the traumatic energy that surrounds me isn't my fault, I feel that I am somehow responsible because I got punished for being:
   - ❖ the whistle blower / honest / myself / courageous
   - ❖ outspoken / different / creative / filled with new ideas
   - ❖ successful / quiet / determined / vocal
   - ❖ open-minded / shallow
   - ❖ alive / having needs / happy / fulfilled
   - ❖ provocative / evocative / powerful / open-minded
   - ❖ naïve / relaxed / brilliant / confident / strong
   - ❖ outshining others / successful / lively / positive
   - ❖ heart-centered / following my heart
   - ❖ peaceful / a humanist / human
   - ❖ trusting / loving / non-judgmental

   Sometimes, I wish that I had been able to remain in the perceived safety of suppressing my true self, so that it's easy to remain part of the tribe.

3) However, the mystical, magical, manifestation energy that we each have, only fully presents itself when we embrace our self-loving truth and act from it. Therefore, when we replace self-blame with self-acceptance, the magic happens. I am now willing to embrace that:
   - ❖ having needs
   - ❖ using my voice
   - ❖ creativity
   - ❖ searching for fulfillment
   - ❖ having fun / living fearlessly
   - ❖ enjoying the little things
   - ❖ being vulnerable / being different
   - ❖ expecting the best
   - ❖ giving and receiving love
   - ❖ intimate connection
   - ❖ knowing that the universe is on my side
   - ❖ speaking my truth
   - ❖ non-judgment
   - ❖ I am the whisperer

   is the path to health and happiness. I now watch as I manifest my beautiful reality from my heart-center of truth.

   Quartz crystal ☺/☺

Compassion Heals Karma

1) I feel unforgivable because I failed to protect:
   - ❖ family member / friend / community / client / student
   - ❖ animal / money
   - ❖ my being / my belongings / my health / my body

   which makes me feel ashamed.

2) This shame point is creating a lack of self-love which is causing me to crave external validation. When I can't get this validation, I crave first thought that comes to mind. Cravings always create heaviness because they can't be fully fulfilled and therefore this heaviness leads to low self-worth.

3) What if I offer unconditional love and complete empathy to me and my genetic line to help release the belief that we need to hold onto shame to keep us on-guard against repeating mistakes. In the end, shame never protects us, it weakens us, and therefore releasing shame is the path to heal all wounds.

4) In summary, holding onto shame creates karma that we work out together within our families and communities. Compassion for every situation resolves karma.

5) With this deep resolve to release shame in order to heal wounds, karma, heaviness, cravings and judgment, I lift my self-worth which helps me find my empathy, leading to forgiveness. When my self-worth is strengthened, it is easy for me to offer love to all, which in turn strengthens their self-worth, which ripples out to all. Without shame, the manifestation of first thought that comes to mind comes with ease.

Quartz crystal ⊘⊘

Dissolving the Angry Mob

Sniff lemon

1) I am in pain because I am afraid of the angry mob. (Go inside and get in touch with who the mob is and its energy.)

2) This pain is residing in my:
   - spine / back / bones
   - feet / toes / ankles / knees / hips / shoulders
   - hands / fingers / elbows / shoulders
   - head / neck / chest / throat
   - lungs / heart / liver / stomach / kidney
   - hair / skin / nails
   - penis / vagina
   - sense organs / body fluids
   - muscles / tendons / ligaments

3) *Close your eyes and feel deeply into the soul of this angry mob to discover the mob's pain.*

4) I now can so clearly see that their pain is the same as mine: my loved-one did not appreciate and honor my loving authenticity.

5) Simply by labeling this deep human pain held by all, my associated fear of:
   - scarcity of: money / time / space / love
   - physical threat / being destroyed in a minute
   - not being able to control my destiny / never getting well
   - exposure/humiliation
   - being controlled/being forced to submit/being enslaved
   - criticism/smugness/disappointing others
   - lack of control which will lead to hurt
   - losing/being a loser/not being included
   - being mischaracterized

   dissolves. My fear of the angry mob was simply covering up my inability to feel safe when I didn't feel love. Because I now choose to honor and appreciate my authentic being, I recognize that I am enough. Because I no longer hide, I am always loved in return.

Serenity tuner ☺☺

Divine Creation

Quartz crystal

1) We are divine creators of our reality. We can manifest anything we want.

2) When I'm not manifesting what I want, it is because I am unconsciously blocking the manifestation. I'm afraid to listen to my heart and manifest first thought that comes to mind because I it might lead to:
   * setting boundaries
   * separating from others
   * taking a risk
   * being too visible
   * setting the record straight
   * setting out on an unrecognizable path
   * making miracles
   * betrayal
   * letting go of (control/things/concepts/people/self-judgment)

   which could:
   * make me unpopular
   * lead to aloneness
   * make me feel exposed
   * put a target on my back
   * disrupt my entire world / feel separated
   * make me too: righteous/outspoken/cocky/ compassionate-less/superior/protective
   * make life so easy that I would forget how to be compassionate to others

3) Following my heart yields free-flow. Holding back yields blocked flow. My blocked flow is actualizing as:
   * things that are hard to heal
   * money that is hard to come by
   * relationships that take too much work
   * unfilled purpose
   * headaches / sleep issues / viruses
   * desperation

4) I now choose to embody the courage and confidence to follow my heart, thereby releasing blocked flow. When I do, I discover that following my heart is actually so much easier and kinder to myself physically, emotionally and spiritually than blocking my flow. I am now manifesting abundance and deeper connection with all.

Divine Love

1) I have created the belief that I need to escape to be relaxed and happy. This belief comes from feeling like I was a disappointment to love-one(s) when I actualized my gifts.

2) In order to avoid criticism, I repress my gifts with:
   - ❖ giving into other's expectations
   - ❖ analysis paralysis
   - ❖ being sick or in pain
   - ❖ money issues
   - ❖ social anxiety / loneliness / relationship issues
   - ❖ unhappiness / unhappy loved-ones
   - ❖ body image
   - ❖ pretending that I'm okay and staying quiet
   - ❖ can't figure out how to market myself
   - ❖ mechanical issues
   - ❖ panic

3) However, due to this lack of actualizing my gifted self, I feel unworthy of (loved-one/God/community/the world)'s love.

4) What if I allowed myself to remember that my authentic gifted being is divine love and a perfect fit for the universe and the more authentic I am, the more content and at peace I am? In my divine authenticity, I naturally love others and they naturally love me in return. And what if now, my loved-ones experience the vibration of my divine love and therefore cannot help but accept my true self in return?

5) I have now created a rejuvenated world of love, laughter, joy and fun.

Quartz crystal ☺☺

Divine Vocation

Sniff wild orange

1) Answer the questions below to identify and gain the courage to discover if you are inhabiting your divine vocation. *(Allow your inner self to answer these questions by going within and listening for the answers.)*

2) Check in with your younger self *(your 10 year old self, your 20 year old self etc.)* to remember what it is you love to do.

   a) Did you shut down your younger self's joy for any reason?

3) Do you do what you love to do as primary work?

   a) Do you judge its value?
   b) Do you need to be in the center of the action to feel valuable?
   c) Do you honor yourself enough to feel worthy and proud of your work?

4) Are you willing to boldly share your divine gifts?

   a) Are you willing to get paid well for sharing?
   b) Are you afraid of disappointing people while doing your work?
   c) Is your work fun?
   d) Are you afraid that your success will intimidate others?
   e) Are you afraid that others won't be there to encourage you, which makes success feel empty?
   f) *If you answered any of questions 4a-e as no, sniff lemon to remember that you when you embrace your divine vocation, then work is joy.*

5) What if you allowed yourself to remember that when you align your work fully with your joyful nature, then you are always valued, supported, cared for and exist in a state of enjoyment?

Quartz crystal ☾☽

Divinely Human

1) If I'm not presenting perfectly, I feel useless, disconnected and non-essential to my (family/community/world).

2) In truth, it is my ego that makes me feel less than, but my heart knows that I'm always divinely human which makes me perfect (even with my flaws) and essential to all communities that I join because I am exactly what is needed.

3) However, I do not feel divinely human because my people didn't care to recognize or acknowledge my talent and/or success because they did not:
    ❖ take care of my (physical/emotional) needs
    ❖ see me as necessary for their joy and happiness
    ❖ want me in their space
    ❖ make themselves available
    ❖ find me to be attractive
    ❖ enjoy my attractiveness
    ❖ like my defiance or independent thinking
    ❖ make my needs a priority
    ❖ believe in me
    ❖ see my new direction coming
    ❖ understand and honor my choices
    ❖ want me to stray from their way of living
    ❖ love me the way I needed to be loved
    ❖ jump into joy with me

4) This oozing wound has caused me to believe that I don't know how to give love because my communities implied that I was unworthy of receiving love (at least in certain times and places). This has left me starving for first thought that comes to mind.

5) What if I remember that simply by giving love to those who choose to receive it is what it means to be divinely human. This is the only factor that truly matters and therefore when I give love, I will always be loved which heals my wounds. And now I know that I am divinely human.

Serenity Tuning Fork

Earth Angels

1) My talent is not recognized by my:
   - ❖ family / friends / acquaintances
   - ❖ myself
   - ❖ teachers / bosses
   - ❖ the general public

   which makes me feel imperfect and unlovable. Then I get down on myself and believe that I'm not quite right for the "job". This energy of worthlessness is actualizing as an addiction to fearful thoughts about:
   - ❖ finances / family / health / commitment

   leading to a sense of overall disappointment.

2) What if others cannot recognize my talent because it disrupts the status quo and disruptions to the status quo can feel existentially threatening?

3) But what if when I actively focus on others with authentic encouragement and praise, I shift the energy for all? Encouragement and praise creates a forcefield of love which raises the vibration for everyone that I come in contact with.

4) And what if inside this forcefield, others are no longer threatened by me and I am not threatened in return because we all see, encourage and praise each other's specialness? And what if when we do, we have all discovered the power of unconditional love to move mountains?

5) What if this act of unconditional love releases all feelings of worthlessness because love feels so important that I choose to become an earth angel spreading love and light throughout the planet?

Quartz crystal ☺/☺

Enlightenment is Bliss

Quartz crystal

1) If I were enlightened, I believe that others might find me to be too:
   ❖ happy / lucky / healthy / relaxed / perfect
   and I might find that I am:
   ❖ bored / unrelatable / smug / compassionless
   ❖ disconnected / unmotivated / lazy / lonely / uninspired
   ❖ righteous / insensitive / unwanted / oppositional
   ❖ irresponsible / too grandiose / too demanding
   and I might end up alone.

2) Therefore, I lower my vibration with energy downers such as:
   ❖ feeling like fraud
   ❖ assuming that I'm broken when something goes wrong
   ❖ not doing something unless it's guaranteed to be above reproach
   ❖ coveting others' popularity, money and/or power
   ❖ lowered compassion
   ❖ feeling unappreciated
   ❖ getting sick / body pain / viruses / infections
   ❖ depression / anxiety / exhaustion
   ❖ headaches / anger / bitterness
   ❖ pessimism / stressed / scared
   ❖ emotional dishonesty and repression
   ❖ difficult: situations/ pets
   ❖ financial stress / lack of success
   ❖ feeling defeated and hopeless
   ❖ situations that are hard to control
   ❖ fighting / jealousy
   ❖ feeling old
   ❖ feeling pushy
   ❖ unconscious sabotage

3) Enlightenment is pure love. What if in this fully loving state things may change, but we would be blissfully happy, serene, healthy, connected, fulfilled and present and we would find each other to be kind, loving, compassionate, helpful, present and fun? Then of course, you would want to be around me, and choose to match my enlightened vibration. Therefore, what if choosing a state of enlightened happiness is risk free, and so I do?

Evolution

Serenity Tuning Fork

1) I easily find myself in the red zone (fear, anxiety, depression, worry, insecurity, anger, grief, frustration, failure, panic, disappointment, sick, compulsive, embarrassment) when I'm triggered.

2) The red zone exists because I don't fully believe that I'm worthwhile and therefore I don't believe that in the face of possible failure, that I'm lovable enough for the benevolent universe to step in and care for me. My belief that I'm not loveable comes from taking a risk and making a mistake when I did it my way (rather than following group norms).

3) *Sit quietly and allow a memory to surface when you took charge and did it your way, but things went wrong, which caused embarrassment.*

4) Embarrassment is often repressed because it's an emotion we hate to feel. Repression leads to energetic blockage actualizing as:

   ❖ headaches / body pain
   ❖ viruses / coughs / infections
   ❖ anxiety / depression / panic
   ❖ money issues / lack of success
   ❖ relationships issues
   ❖ too much work

5) The green zone of safety and happiness is easily accessed when I embrace the truth that doing it my way is the only way to find fulfillment and that I am lovable even when my way is imperfect.

6) From this perspective, course corrections leading to happiness, health, abundance and fulfillment naturally actualize from the vibration of my heart and I am at peace.

Flower of Life

Sniff lemon

1) My authentic gifted being is divine love and a perfect fit for the perfect universe. The universe becomes imperfect when we believe in the construct of scarcity. In this construct, our egos are always scared and then we fight over scarce resources through conflict and wars, yielding more scarcity.

2) This construct of scarcity comes from the wounding event of the scarcity of love from first thing that comes to mind. This construct of lack is deeper when this wound has not been resolved, creating space for addictions, illness, avoidance and/or dysfunction to fill the void.

3) Within scarcity thinking scenarios arise:
   ❖ Self-importance takes hold and we believe that we have the right to grab – which starts wars. This energy craves validation and holds back on appreciation.
   ❖ I hide my needs so I don't get punished.
   ❖ I exist in a state of embarrassment and/or fear.
   ❖ I am constantly trying to prove my rightness.
   ❖ The need to be consequential so that I'm worthy of attention and resources.
   ❖ I need to be seen to be worthy.

4) What if I remember that my love is so strong that it fills all voids? And from this love, I gather others to love, naturally focusing on appreciation of myself and others. In this new state of love and appreciation, I feel abundance around me, and scarcity and war dissipate.

The flower of love's creative and wholistic energy powers this protocol so that giving love naturally releases fear. From this space we utilize our gifts to create peace and happiness and our energy is boundless.

Serenity Tuning Fork

Freedom

Sniff lemon & wild orange

1) I am embarrassed that I can't control my:
   - ❖ body function/illness/mind/thoughts/actions
   - ❖ aging/deterioration/health
   - ❖ loved-ones/pets
   - ❖ weight/appearance/addictions/desires/habits
   - ❖ finances/empty calendar/what you are willing to pay me
   - ❖ cleanliness/neediness/messiness/carelessness
   - ❖ perception of my value
   - ❖ energy/actions/anger/responses/moods/laziness
   - ❖ weaknesses/mistakes/messiness/failures
   - ❖ personality/loud voice/pushiness/preferences
   - ❖ environment/country/community/religion/world
   - ❖ what you think of me/need to exist
   - ❖ emotions/needs/need for attention
   - ❖ rocking the boat/non-traditional ways
   - ❖ essence (who I am)/quirks/desires

2) What if lack of control isn't the problem, but embarrassment is the problem. Feeling embarrassed is an emotion that we hate to feel so I squash it with:
   - ❖ blaming, anger & vindictiveness
   - ❖ defensiveness/disappointment
   - ❖ numbing addictions/over eating/restricting
   - ❖ fear/phobia/paranoia
   - ❖ exhaustion/lack of focus/lack of success
   - ❖ obsessions/compulsions/micromanagement
   - ❖ hiding due to fear of exposure/jealousy/rudeness
   - ❖ trying to be perfect/avoidance
   - ❖ illness/pain/teeth issues
   - ❖ stressful situations
   - ❖ absent mindedness

3) The solution is simple. The answer is the self-acceptance that comes from honestly recognizing our strengths and weaknesses without blaming ourselves or others. Then, we can give ourselves a break by accepting who we are and where we are at. This is the absolute FREEDOM that comes from a truthful narrative.

4) Once we are free, embarrassment fades, and we naturally live life fully. I am now free and easy.

Fueling my Bliss

Serenity Tuning Fork

1) I hold onto not healing first thing that comes to mind because healing means releasing guilt about first things that comes to mind. I'm afraid to release guilt because I am afraid that without guilt, I might lose my attachment to caring about first things that comes to mind.

2) What if in this magical world that we are creating, we are always there for each other and naturally use our gifts to help others? And what if we don't have to experience pain, illness and toxicity to be motivated to discover solutions?

3) And what if I'm blocking the experience of this heavenly existence because I'm afraid of the state of blissful kindness because:
    ❖ I don't trust others to respect and take care of me when my guard is down
    ❖ others might (shame/reject/take advantage of) me when my guard is down
    ❖ there would be no suffering and therefore, I wouldn't be worthy of love
    ❖ one of us might get hurt when my guard is down
    ❖ I can't hold onto my coping mechanisms when my guard is down
    ❖ I won't have an excuse to check out
    ❖ there would be no reason to reach out for care
    ❖ I wouldn't relate to your struggle and therefore I wouldn't be able to access compassion
    ❖ I need to have someone to blame so I don't surface my own shame
    ❖ I might fly away from my loved ones because special connections wouldn't be important to me because I would connect to everyone
    ❖ others might not relate to my bliss
    ❖ I would be bored and disconnected
    ❖ because difficulties bring out others compassion
    But in fact, a state of deeply loving and respectful connections is what fuels our bliss.

4) I choose to release my guilt and therefore I choose to release suffering by harnessing the loving energy inside of me to manifest love all around me.

Quartz crystal

Happy, Healthy and Alive

1) I am not achieving:
   - good health
   - loving relationships
   - life affirming work
   - financial freedom

   because I exist in a pattern of overwork, overthinking and stress.

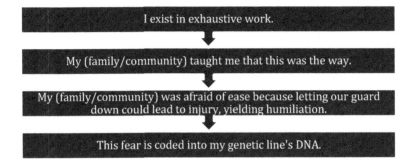

I exist in exhaustive work.

↓

My (family/community) taught me that this was the way.

↓

My (family/community) was afraid of ease because letting our guard down could lead to injury, yielding humiliation.

↓

This fear is coded into my genetic line's DNA.

2) Exhaustive work is so punishing that I consciously choose another way.

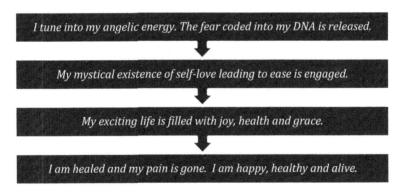

I tune into my angelic energy. The fear coded into my DNA is released.

↓

My mystical existence of self-love leading to ease is engaged.

↓

My exciting life is filled with joy, health and grace.

↓

I am healed and my pain is gone. I am happy, healthy and alive.

Quartz crystal

Heaven on Earth

1) I resent <small>first thought that comes to mind</small> because (he/she/they/it) didn't serve my need for relaxation. What if instead, I recognize that I am the only one who can serve my need for relaxation? And what if I have been afraid to take ownership of creating relaxation because resentment is the shield that helps me blame something or someone other than me. However, needing a shield creates inauthenticity which actualizes as:
   - ❖ viruses / allergies
   - ❖ lack of success

2) It is very hard to let go of the need for a shield because our egos are deathly afraid of criticism and being blamed. *In order to release the ego's fears, enter a rest your palms face up and breathe deeply. Check to see if you can feel heaviness, tingling or warmth emanating from your hands. These sensations are the indicator that you have entered the energy of heaven on earth.*

3) Within heaven on earth we naturally love ourselves. Within self-love the ego drops it's fear of criticism and blame because *(dowse as many as apply):*
   - ❖ we no longer believe our negative thoughts
   - ❖ we recognize that only love is real
   - ❖ we no longer judge ourselves and others (rather, we encourage)
   - ❖ we naturally release our defenses
   - ❖ we no longer need to feel in control so stress is gone
   - ❖ we don't experience feeling threatened
   - ❖ we feel our confidence rising and we expect success
   - ❖ we are 100% comfortable in our authentic expression
   - ❖ we fully trust self, our decisions, our beauty and our vision
   - ❖ righteous discourse is gone
   - ❖ we experience grace and kindness all around us and therefore we always fit in
   - ❖ we recognize that we have complete agency over our life
   - ❖ pain and dis-ease resolve as our body regenerates to its healthiest form
   - ❖ our manifestation is always aligned with our heart

   Within this ego release, we now have the guts to trust our instinctual self and discover that we are living in heaven on earth.

Serenity Tuning Fork

Hero, Victim, Villain

1) Today, I am the victim, you are the villain and someone else is the hero. This triangle has created chaos so none of us feel the need take ownership of the chaos. This chaos is actualizing as:
   - ❖ headaches / fevers / dehydration / dry eyes
   - ❖ viruses / infections / cough
   - ❖ lack
   - ❖ war / poverty / political fighting / mischaracterization
   - ❖ mechanical issues

2) In order to balance this cycle, I embrace that in any dramatic circumstance, I can be the victim, villain and/or hero. In truth, I always want to be the hero. However, as I try to control the situation while taking the hero's role, it often falls apart and I can be the victim (*why did this happen to me?*) and the villain (*was I self-absorbed in this situation?*). The healing is to compassionately recognize everyone's struggle, sending love to all including myself.

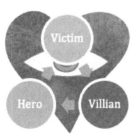

3) In my state of complete compassion for all, I have woken to the new consciousness. I have been afraid of this consciousness because I believed that living in absolute bliss would separate me from my loved ones and I would be alone. However, within complete compassion, I am never separate. Instead, I am the energy that everyone else needs to elevate to their enlightened state. We are one, we are whole and we are love and in this state we are always heroes.

Quartz crystal ᕙᕗ

Honoring my Soul

Quartz crystal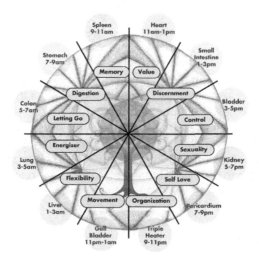

1) <small>Fill in with unsolved problem</small> exists because I feel that I don't deserve success because of my ugly, yet repressed feelings that I am a <small>close your eyes and speak all words that come into your head</small>. *(Surfacing these emotions sets you free.)*

2) I'm ready to recognize that I hold onto the belief that I'm not worthy, as a form of constant punishment, to help me overcome my weaknesses in order to achieve success. This is the ego's path to success.

3) I am ready to recognize that instead, if I honor my vulnerability, then I achieve true success. This is a sacred truth because honoring vulnerability yields authenticity and only within authenticity can we achieve the type of success that makes happy. **This is the heart's path to success.**

4) *With clear quartz in hand, spiral in and then out over truth clock below (to balance the meridian cycle) to create the shift into honoring vulnerability which is the key to sharing my soul's greatness with the world.*

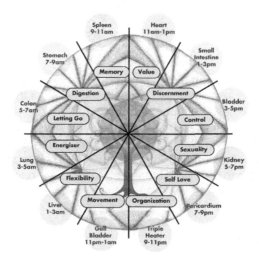

Serenity Tuning Fork

Humanness Yields Success

1) I feel like I can't make any mistakes in my relationships because I might get criticized. This potential for criticism brings me back to a memory of disdain leading to rejection. *Close your eyes, breathe deeply to allow the memory of rejection to surface.*

2) Because of this weighty unprocessed emotional complex, I have unconsciously created fear constructs around others seeing me as wrong when I authentically actualize:
   ❖ a lot of money / success
   ❖ my abundant way of life
   ❖ what love means to me / good friends

3) My fear construct actualizes as:
   ❖ walking on eggshells
   ❖ imagining the worst
   ❖ believing that I'm a loser
   ❖ afraid to stand-up for myself
   ❖ needing validation / feeling like disappointment
   ❖ avoidance / invisibility / setting the bar low
   ❖ not trusting (the universe's flow/that my needs are valid
   ❖ a lack of self-respect
   ❖ anxiety / depression
   ❖ bad health
   ❖ feeling (unsuccessful / unworthy / inadequate)
   ❖ tricky relationships
   ❖ anger / suspicion
   ❖ perfectionism / procrastination
   ❖ not having enough of what I need (money/friends/work…)
   My fear construct holds me back in both personal relationships and professional success.

4) The magic happens when this memory and the associated fear-based construct is identified. Whether the judgment of the earlier event is accurate or not, I now recognize that the rejecting response has already happened so there's nothing more to be afraid of.

5) Once the originating event is uncovered and explored, then the fear construct releases. Without fear, I don't judge myself for my choices. Instead, I allow for my humanness, which eases the emotional load, leading to personal and professional success as I manifest health, wealth and happiness.

I AM a Mystical Magical Magician

1) I feel that I did not get my need for (care/encouragement/fun/ love/relaxation) met by loved-one and therefore I feel (alone/dampened/burdened/unpopular/scrutinized/stupid/ wrong). Therefore achieving self-empowerment feels out of reach.

2) What if I remember that I am a mystical magical magician and that I can always naturally manifest all that I need simply through self-love? And what if self-love can be achieved by identifying that I feel ashamed of first thought that comes to mind?

3) What if I remember that everyone carries the shame that comes with attempting to fill love-voids? And what if I make a commitment to believe in myself and others even if at times we are hurtful? And what if believe that the goodness of humanity fills the love-void and then I can feel the love?

4) And what if in my new-found experience of believing in humanity, I am always compassionate towards the obstacles and sorrow that we have gone through? And what if this compassion is so strong that I can't judge another's pain or life choices? And what if without judgment, love is easy and my mystical magical magician takes the lead?

5) My mystical magical magician experiences:
    *   everyone and everything as love
    *   gratitude, appreciation and joy are our natural states
    *   through self-love we create the abundant world of our dreams and we stop hurting each other
    *   a life of absolute success
    *   a loving world

6) Take a moment to visualize what the abundant and loving world looks and feels like and revel in the possibility of it all.

I AM Celebrating Me

1) I can't release the nagging feeling that in order to be
   successful, I need to follow the codes of my:
   - family / friends / teacher / profession / institution
   - religion / group / nationality / gender
   - partner / community / profession / professionals
   - social group
   - society / humanity / people in charge

2) Even though these codes can sometimes feel harsh, not
   following a code makes me feel like I'm doing something
   wrong and I'm scared of getting ostracized.   Therefore I
   perceive that I must follow these codes and I catastrophize a
   horrific outcome that might occur if I don't follow community
   norms.

3) I now recognize that I have been conditioned by harsh codes
   that don't celebrate me. In truth harsh codes harden me,
   and therefore I haven't been able to see my clear path to
   success.

4) To clear my path to success, I run all codes through my
   heart and only accept those that celebrate me. (Anything
   that causes me to beat myself up or question myself isn't
   truth.) However, accepting only that which aligns with my
   loving truth releases my painful:
   - OCD / depression / anxiety
   - loneliness / starvation
   - lack of: love / romance / money / sex / fun
   - body / mind / spirit / soul
   - viruses / cough / infections
   - upside down decision making
   and I am celebrating me and I am free.

Quartz crystal

I AM Consequential

1) I lost my sense of pride because _{loved-one} could not show pride for my authentic:
    - ❖ body/beauty
    - ❖ love/trust
    - ❖ intellect
    - ❖ boundaries
    - ❖ assertiveness/determination
    - ❖ persistence/resilience/work ethic
    - ❖ success/talent/gifts
    - ❖ creations
    - ❖ spirit/spunk/joy
    - ❖ power/voice
    - ❖ creative pursuits/fresh ideas
    - ❖ relaxed nature/adaptability
    - ❖ intimacy
    - ❖ sexuality
    - ❖ value/desires/identity
    - ❖ leadership
    - ❖ presence
    - ❖ individuality/uniqueness/philosophy

    because the perception of a lack of perfection in these areas (either for my loved-one or me) caused embarrassing exposure which depleted my self-pride.

2) However the lack of my loved-one's pride makes me feel completely inconsequential. This feeling is so painful that I attempt to distract myself with:
    - ❖ keeping myself small
    - ❖ numbing addictions
    - ❖ overwhelm/catastrophizing
    - ❖ stressful situations
    - ❖ chronic: illness/pain/viruses
    - ❖ dysfunction
    - ❖ trying too hard/socially avoidant
    - ❖ anxiety/depression/nervousness
    - ❖ narcissism
    - ❖ analysis paralysis/obsession
    - ❖ politics

3) This fear based programming is deprogrammed by choosing to be enthusiastically oneself at all times. Authentic enthusiasm always leads to finding the place in which I am always authentically consequential.

Quartz crystal ☺☺

I AM Effortless Creation

Sniff wild orange

1) Are you ready to actualize effortless creation?

2) If the answer is yes or no, the follow-up steps are the same because effortless creation is our natural state of existence. When we make choices based on what we love, rather than based on fear and other's expectations, we block our effortless creative force.

3) However I sometimes make choices based on fear and on other's expectations, because I am afraid of:
   - ❖ ostracism
   - ❖ criticism or judgment
   - ❖ painful consequences
   - ❖ getting disrespected
   - ❖ getting hurt / feeling disloyal / losing you
   - ❖ not listening to another's opinion and then being wrong
   - ❖ other's opinion that I'm selfish, wrong, unappreciative, irresponsible and thoughtless
   - ❖ feeling foolish
   - ❖ feeling like the price of making a mistake is too high and I can't recover
   - ❖ trusting my intuition when it's different than yours
   - ❖ living in self-doubt and regret
   - ❖ publicly crashing and burning
   - ❖ "be careful what you wish for"
   - ❖ letting someone down / leaving others behind
   - ❖ my independent nature might create suspicion
   - ❖ letting my guard down / being out of control
   - ❖ that the right choice isn't available to me
   - ❖ group think righteousness
   - ❖ my success creating unwanted consequences

4) What if a universal truth is that when we make decisions from the heart, even if they cause disruption or require course corrections, then we are proclaiming "I am self-love" (rather than proclaiming I am scared). When our actions show self-love to the universe, then the universe responds to our heart and we create our magical, wonderful, playful world. And then we become effortless creation.

Serenity Tuning Fork

I AM Enlightenment

Sniff wild orange

1) My ego tells me that decisions are important because my ego doesn't want to make mistakes that have consequences or make me look foolish.

2) My heart tells me that decisions don't matter; living life matters. And if the "wrong" decision is made, course corrections from the heart will always yield happiness.

3) Because I'm not ready to believe this concept, I stress about my decisions. The biggest decision that I'm stressing about is first thought that comes to mind. Making the wrong decision feels so important because I believe that it could lead to unhappiness. I now operate in a space of fear regarding decisions.

4) In order to avoid unhappiness, I put great weight around my decisions. This weight creates a body blockage actualizing as:
   ❖ viruses / infections / headaches / congestion / cough
   ❖ weight gain / disordered eating
   ❖ digestive issues
   ❖ addiction
   ❖ lack of: connected intimacy / joy

5) What if I have the equation wrong? What if I simply let my heart manifest the well-lit path to joy? Then the direction and need for course corrections are clear. And what if allowing my heart to lead always creates transcendent joy and releases the blocks that impede body function?

6) And what if I trust this sacred truth because in fact I usually allow my heart to lead, and things only cause stress when I lead from fear while ignoring my heart? And what if I've just chosen enlightenment?

I AM Free

Quartz crystal

5) I've stopped believing in my:
   - ❖ leadership
   - ❖ self-love / self-care
   - ❖ gifts / potential / value / purpose
   - ❖ creative spirit / individuality
   - ❖ genius / knowhow
   - ❖ healership / inspirational vision

   because _{loved-one}'s insecurities prefer it when I stay small. I "help" myself stay small with:
   - ❖ sickness / disease / viruses / body pain
   - ❖ chronic conditions / breathing issues / congestion / cough
   - ❖ addiction / weight / denial
   - ❖ money issues
   - ❖ feeling like I don't belong / feeling unpopular
   - ❖ unfinished projects / over-focusing on others
   - ❖ war and destruction
   - ❖ feeling undeserving
   - ❖ objections and excuses
   - ❖ lack of sleep / lack of exercise
   - ❖ anxiety / depression / dread
   - ❖ perfectionism leading to self-criticism and blame
   - ❖ addiction / shame and blame of self and others
   - ❖ diminishing my voice
   - ❖ resentment / revenge fantasies / negativity
   - ❖ living in madness / powerless situations
   - ❖ stagnation / headaches
   - ❖ toxicity
   - ❖ memory issues / absent mindedness
   - ❖ toggling between tired and grumpy or bored and useless

6) What if just for today, I give myself permission to be enthusiastically myself, which always leads to strength and success, even in the face of backlash and punishment? And what if my authentically enthusiastic energy creates a forcefield of love that is so strong that other's insecurities cannot penetrate or bring me down?

7) And what if I'm further emboldened to be myself because I see through other's insecurities and therefore I'm no longer scared of punishment? And what if my authentic enthusiasm always releases other's hold over me and I am now free?

I AM Friends with my Best Life

Hold quartz crystal

1) I have resisted living my best life because I believe that my best life always means:
   ❖ being happy while accepting loss with ease
   ❖ being popular while being authentic
   ❖ being driven while being gentle
   ❖ being optimistic without being cocky
   ❖ being brave and beyond reproach at the same time
   ❖ being bold and never having regrets at the same time
   ❖ being perky, energetic and hardworking while maintaining my freedom
   ❖ enjoying down-time without getting bored
   ❖ being flawless beyond reproach
   ❖ being kind while maintaining limits
   ❖ being approved of while approving of myself
   ❖ being special without feeling grandiose
   ❖ being endlessly patient while still having enough time for me
   ❖ making time for me and you
   ❖ making choices that are good for me, but you also like these same choices
   ❖ being respectful and powerful at the same time
   ❖ being carefree and careful at the same time
   ❖ being visible and quietly humble at the same time
   ❖ being selfless, kind and fulfilled all at once
   ❖ being active and accomplished, yet relaxed

   but I don't believe that I can achieve this state of perfection. Therefore, I close off parts of myself with:
   ❖ sadness / depression / isolation
   ❖ anxiety / lack of confidence / micromanagement
   ❖ scarcity / difficult loved-ones or pets
   ❖ analysis paralysis / regret / fear of regret / hyper-vigilance
   ❖ chronic pain / illness / viruses / addiction
   ❖ restlessness / sleeplessness / hyperactivity
   ❖ strong opinions that offend others
   ❖ can't remember details / can't focus on the big picture

   all leading to self-absorption and a lack of presence and forward movement.

2) What if living my best life just means being friends with myself and therefore choosing to boldly follow my heart-felt pleasure and then the rest simply falls into place—not with perfection but with authenticity accompanied by the power to love my mistakes and failures because they show me the way? And what if when I'm friends with my best life, then boldly living and loving is effortless creation?
   Serenity Tuning Fork ◎/◎

I AM my Higher Self

Hold quartz crystal

1) Because I perceived that I would be rejected by
   (family/friends/community/peers/ancestors/humanity) for my:
   ❖ sexual preference/gender preference
   ❖ vocation/knowledge/power/extraordinary gifts
   ❖ partner choice/tastes/lack of perfection
   ❖ recognition that everything that happens can brings us to greater love
   ❖ adventures/risks/point of view/playfulness
   ❖ religious choice/spiritual grace/attractiveness/positivity
   ❖ understanding that love is all there is and the only thing that creates true healing

   I hide myself with the help of:
   ❖ pain/disease/virus/infection/allergies
   ❖ judgment/feeling inconsiderate/feeling judged
   ❖ frightened/insecurity/self-loathing
   ❖ lack of intimacy/fighting/manipulation blame
   ❖ stress/scarcity/irritability/agitation
   ❖ addiction/unrequited love/hyperactivity
   ❖ sleeplessness/exhaustion/circadian rhythms off
   ❖ lack of abundance/sticky problems/world problems
   ❖ isolation/unfeeling/difficult loved-ones or pets
   ❖ weight/aging/deterioration/worn out
   ❖ disappointment/betrayal/feeling victimized
   ❖ anxiety/depression/emotional dishonesty
   ❖ imbalances/micromanagement/obsession
   ❖ make a joke out of everything

   I make this choice to hide because hiding protects me from the heartbreak of being unsupported and ostracized and this heartbreak feels too painful to bear.

2) But what if living authentically, which means living as self-love, always creates the life of my dreams even if there is some disruption and heartbreak along the way?

3) In this state of authentic love, I become one with my higher self and my mind and body merge with spiritual lightness and joy. Choosing authenticity becomes easy and is worth it, always, and so I do! I am now effortless creation.

I AM the I AM

Hold quartz crystal

1) I am afraid to ask for my need for first thought that comes to mind to be met because my need for care and compassion was not met by unavailable and unresponsive (parent/loved one/world/ friend/body processes/community/workers/ professional/ God/faith/boss/helpers/strangers/universe/profession/ mind/body/teacher/friends/lover/employer/clients/medicine).

2) I now only trust me to be the doer. Therefore I obsessively:
   - overwork / fix / micro-manage / acquiesce / share
   - overthink / overanalyze / second guess / avoid
   - dominate / demand flexibility / conceal / over-complicate
   - defend and deflect
   - disconnect / choose not to commit
   - avoid / hide inside my pain body
   - am super-efficient
   - am a perfectionist
   - procrastinate / stay small / shut down production

   These coping skills have been somewhat effective in filling my needs. However the fear of the unfulfilled need-void has deepened the void, because my ego doesn't trust the quantum field of possible solutions and wants to fill the void in very specific ways, making it hard for the universe to fulfill that script. Therefore my coping skills have created scarcity, lack of trust, pain and exhaustion.

3) What if I remember and acknowledge that I am the I AM, simply by being and having a wish. Therfore, I have the absolute ability to create and heal in an instant anything that I desire from the heart. I now trust the vast universe to fulfill my needs because everyone and everything is responsive, caring and loving to me. And then I easily have the space to be responsive to your needs in return.

4) I ask the universe to fulfill my wishes as I trust the actualization of my wish to present itself in the best and most beautiful form for me. I now see my world as a magical and whimsical playground. I don't experience problems.

Sniff lemon

I Am the Main Character

Serenity Tuning Fork

1) I know that if I give when it feels like love, then my existence is life-affirming. I also know that if I choose to hold back my loving gifts because of my fear of an unloving response, then I experience lack forming as the construct of:
    - ❖ pain conditions
    - ❖ money issues
    - ❖ unfulfilling work
    - ❖ relationship drama
    - ❖ stressful interactions
    - ❖ ugliness
    - ❖ always feeling the need to apologize
    - ❖ indecisiveness
    - ❖ social interactions
    - ❖ self-loathing
    - ❖ compared and I lose

2) I recognize that I can only give from my heart when I first give love to me. Giving love to me is the most important step to self-empowerment. Although scary, I choose to recognize my value and share my gifts with those who enjoy what I have to offer, because self-empowerment creates miraculous abundance and the experience of floating with life. When I do, lack does not exist within loving self-empowerment.

3) It is not possible for me to experience life any longer as the disowned outsider because sharing my love makes me the main character in my story. As the loving protagonist, others gather around me, filling my voids with love, because my space is so warm, helpful and inviting, we are finally free to love again.

Sniff wild orange

I AM the Vibration of Success

1) I strive for success but I can't seem to truly get there. My lack of success stems from a time when I experienced success but it felt like loved-one was not there to acknowledge or support me. This created a massive void in my heart which I never want to feel again so I do everything I can do to resist the quiet of being alone with my success through:
   ❖ tics and/or uncontrollable urges that are always by my side
   ❖ the need to grab recognition however I can, often in the form of being a mess or getting in trouble
   ❖ perfectionism and high expectations as the excuse to beat myself up making it hard to succeed
   ❖ a demeaning partner so I always feel like a failure
   ❖ fatigue / depression / anxiety / headaches
   ❖ regrets and analysis paralysis so I'm stuck in the past.
   ❖ trauma which fills me with pain
   ❖ having an addiction which blurs the emptiness
   ❖ "buying" connections with my generosity
   ❖ social anxiety which helps me avoid empty conversations
   ❖ chronic pain and illness
   ❖ accidents and injuries preventing an easy flow
   ❖ constant financial stress
   ❖ weight issues yielding insecurity
   ❖ panic and other forms of mental illness
   ❖ uncooperative pets and children
   ❖ spinning
   ❖ headaches of all kinds
   ❖ unpopularity

2) What if I give up my fear of being alone in my success, because I am able at this moment of clarity to choose to celebrate my own success? And what if my celebration is so contagious that others always want to join me because it's fun and celebrating each other is our natural state of being? And what if I can make this choice because it's what I have desired my whole life and resistance is now futile because I am the vibration of success? And what if I've now created a fulfilling and successful life shared with others?

Quartz crystal ☺☺

I AM Vibration Happy

1) When I am authentically happy, but _{loved-one} cannot get there, this loved-one can punish my happiness with heartbreaking:
   * betrayal
   * jealousy / playing the victim / poutiness
   * mischaracterizations / gaslighting / blaming
   * anger / fighting / yelling / war / attacks / torture
   * disapproval / guilt trips / manipulative / unavailable
   * desertion / criticism / indignity / mocking / torment

2) I unconsciously allow the chronic symptoms of:
   * viruses / coughs / congestion
   * weight / constant hunger / no appetite
   * body pain / headaches
   * money issues / work dissatisfaction
   * depression / anxiety / addiction
   * Lyme / Covid
   * sadness
   * hormonal imbalances
   * family stress / pet stress / accidents

   to persist as they help me manage the punishment quotient because they make me feel less guilty for my success and happiness while lowering my happy vibrations.

3) What if I allow my vibration to return to "vibration happy" by enjoying my luck without feeling guilty for all that life has given me? And what if I acknowledge that I have created my "luck" from my happy vibrations, and that this "luck" is available to all of us when we make course corrections to create happiness?

4) I am now determined to make course corrections to help me create my happy vibration, even though others cannot get there yet. My first course correction is to stop yielding my happiness to a punishing loved-one. And what if when I remain steadfast in my choice to be happy, it's so infectious that others join me? Then our happiness spreads and we have discovered how to create happiness with all.

I AM Who I AM

1) Our natural state is to know that we are kind, smart and important and therefore our value and self-worth are intact. We feel necessary and special and are celebrating our fulfilling and loving life.

2) However, I was wounded by loved-one who made me feel:
   - ❖ left out / unwanted / like I didn't fit in / not enough
   - ❖ untalented / lacking comprehension / like I was failing
   - ❖ not prioritized / not appreciated / irrelevant
   - ❖ not (understood/respected/wanted/needed)
   - ❖ unattractive / like a bother / embarrassed
   - ❖ inconsiderate / shameful / wrong

   Self-doubt and a lack of self-worth set in and I protect my ego with:
   - ❖ perfectionism / the quest for popularity
   - ❖ lying / dishonesty / sneakiness / denial
   - ❖ panic / possessiveness
   - ❖ sickness / pain / exhaustion
   - ❖ respiratory infections
   - ❖ a broken will

   I now need constant validation to feel good about myself, which can be impossible to achieve.

3) What if I recognized that my lack of self-worth is an illusion and it is simply my woundedness that makes me feel unnecessary and unimportant? And what if I can access my unlimited source and recognize that my being is exactly what the planet needs at this time because I am naturally celebrating myself because I am who I am!

Quartz crystal ☺/☺

I AM Worthy

1) I haven't been able to manifest <small>first thought that comes to mind</small> because I am not allowing myself to express my worth.

2) What if I'm able to treasure the desires that come from my heart, because I AM the person who knows me the best? Therefore, I know that believing in what's best for me, is the perspective that counts the most. Believing in me, opens the path to success, elevating my self-worth, actualizing as the energy of love all around me. *Walk through cycle below to shift into self-worth through self-belief.*

I Am Worthy Cycle

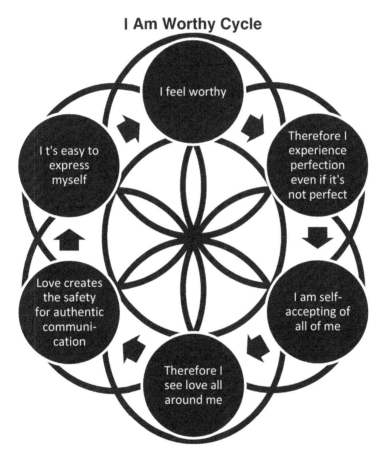

3) Within complete self-acceptance, I embody authentic expression and, my world is healed as my dreams naturally manifest.

I Believe in Myself

1) I feel like I can't trust first thought that comes to mind. Trust is a mirror and when I don't trust myself, I'm surrounded by others that I can't always trust. I'm starting to realize that I don't trust my gifted:
   - ❖ reliability
   - ❖ accountability / memory
   - ❖ integrity (being true to self)
   - ❖ generosity
   - ❖ intelligence
   - ❖ confidence
   - ❖ abilities
   - ❖ new ideas
   - ❖ power
   - ❖ leadership
   - ❖ ability to heal
   - ❖ clarity
   - ❖ connection
   - ❖ the future / the past

   because loved-one(s) did not encourage me to believe in myself this way. This lack of self-trust makes it hard for me to believe in myself enough to:
   - ❖ set firm boundaries / support my opinions
   - ❖ be self-supporting
   - ❖ stop worrying
   - ❖ handle other's demands
   - ❖ be emotionally honest about hard situations
   - ❖ know that I can succeed
   - ❖ feel admired and desired
   - ❖ welcome you in
   - ❖ stay in touch / be in your presence / share my energy
   - ❖ believe that I'm worthy of attention
   - ❖ be vulnerable / relax my guard / let you in
   - ❖ break the rules

2) What if this recognition is enough for me to recognize that my insecurities are illusions and my gifted being is truth? When I allow this truth to be true, then I trust myself. When I trust myself, then the energy of the people that I surround myself with, lifts to meet my vibration. Now we are all trustworthy, and our lives become successful and easy.

Sniff wild orange

I Choose to Accept Myself

1) Because I was condemned by _{loved-one} for being:
   ❖ overweight
   ❖ lazy / undisciplined
   ❖ not mindful of rules / difficult / disobedient
   ❖ open minded / different
   ❖ not religious / not God fearing / immoral
   ❖ true to my identity / inquisitive
   ❖ (smarter/more knowledgeable/more attractive) than you
   ❖ physically challenged / learning challenged
   ❖ sick / needy
   ❖ easy going / going with the flow
   ❖ kind and generous
   ❖ thoughtless / unkind / not generous enough
   ❖ irresponsible

   it has made me scared for _{loved-one} and me if we display these characteristics. Therefore I hide my presence with overwhelming:
   ❖ procrastination
   ❖ addiction
   ❖ isolation / aggression / anger
   ❖ failing / lack of success
   ❖ clutter
   ❖ setting high goals that I cannot achieve
   ❖ anxiety / depression / panic
   ❖ exhaustion
   ❖ body pain / headaches
   ❖ money issues / expenses / projects
   ❖ family issues / pet issues / stress
   ❖ not feeling like I can hold my own
   ❖ perfectionism which I can't maintain

2) What if I remember that I can be imperfect and perfect at the same time? It's actually accepting my needs, desires, personality and imperfections that make me perfect.

3) Self-acceptance happens naturally when I give myself space and grace. There is no down-side to self-acceptance. Self-acceptance releases fear and shame leading to health, wealth and happiness. The choice to self-accept is now so obvious, that I choose to make this choice, always.

Quartz crystal ☺/☺

I Matter

Serenity Tuning Fork

1) I cannot manifest _{first thought that comes to mind}, even though I have tried. This lack persists because I am afraid of this manifestation because I feel that celebrating success would mean celebrating alone, which makes me feel like I don't matter.

2) The fear of feeling empty and alone when I achieve success has caused me to disengage my internal compass. This disengagement has led to:
   ❖ not trusting my decisions
   ❖ seeking a black and white philosophy so I can follow the rules so I don't get into trouble
   ❖ limiting my body with pain and sickness
   ❖ limiting my mind
   ❖ illness/memory issues/learning deficits
   ❖ nasty self-talk/limiting beliefs
   ❖ chaotic situations
   ❖ accidents/emergencies/scary moments
   ❖ feeling solution-less
   ❖ lack of money
   ❖ lack of identity
   ❖ feeling unfulfilled
   ❖ feeling inconsequential
   ❖ feeling lost

3) The healing is to enthusiastically and generously trust and honor my internal compass with the recognition that my compass is aligned to my heart. Trusting my compass may cause disruption, but always rewards me with enlightened discoveries that show me that the abundant universe is on my side.

4) Now, my fear of being empty and alone has been replaced with peaceful self-acceptance, yielding strong knowingness that I Matter! In the state of I Matter, viruses cannot enter my body because my body does not accept that which is not of love.

Sniff wild orange

Integrating into Peace on Earth

Serenity Tuning Fork

1) I align with the tribe of <small>state first "tribe" that comes to mind</small> in order to:
   - ❖ protect resources
   - ❖ support my philosophy
   - ❖ feel at home in a community
   - ❖ strengthen my identity
   - ❖ generate sympathy for each other
   - ❖ feel worthy of complaining
   - ❖ diminish my power so I can blend in
   - ❖ hide and protect my time and space
   - ❖ be the victim so I can feel righteous

   but this alignment splinters me from the rest of the world and creates a fight over resources because we are entrenched in the belief that resources are scarce.

2) What if I remember that all tribes are part of the whole because each tribe represents a part of each of us that yearns for connection, love and security? And what if our tribes remember that resources aren't scarce; it's simply the fight over them that wastes resources and causes scarcity?

3) Once the belief in scarcity releases, we give ourselves permission to embrace all parts of our personality, interests and needs without fighting for our right to be who we are. In this new-found energy of wholeness, we seamlessly connect with everything. The need to disconnect and fight has now disappeared and abundance abounds.

4) We now deeply understand that in our authenticity we are an integral part of everything. Therefore we never forget our worth and self-acceptance is our norm. We are at peace and the world is at peace.

Sniff wild orange

I've Got This

1) I would feel more peaceful and joyful if I created first thought that they would like to create. However, I resist creating this because I perceive that: *(dowse one or more)*
   - ❖ success may cause insecure loved-ones to deflate me
   - ❖ success may cause me to abandon others because of my lack of time and space
   - ❖ if it comes easy to me, I might not relate to other's failure and pain (and others might find me to lack humility)
   - ❖ if everything came easy I wouldn't need God and I would miss the relationship
   - ❖ I love adventure and easy success takes removes the adventure
   - ❖ true success requires me to embrace my ideals and I'm afraid that others would reject these ideals

2) What if I know down deep that success creates greater connection to everyone's hearts, rather than abandonment? And what if this knowingness regenerates my mind, body, spirit and soul. And what if now the voice in my head that says, "success is scary" is replaced with the knowingness that "I've got this". I am now good with myself and therefore I know that no one can, or wants to, take me down.

It's a Valid Concern, Let's Talk About It

Serenity Tuning Fork

1) It's very hard for me to hear your concern because it may:
   - ❖ cost me money
   - ❖ take time / make it worse
   - ❖ ruin my plans / ruin my fun / make me feel bad
   - ❖ cause me: to miss out / be left out
   - ❖ make me look bad / ruin my reputation
   - ❖ feel like criticism
   - ❖ make me feel like a fool / make me feel like a bad person
   - ❖ makes me feel sad and hopeless / break my heart
   - ❖ feel like the solution makes it harder for me
   - ❖ be inconvenient / be hard to fix
   - ❖ impose on me
   - ❖ put me on path that I'm not interested in
   - ❖ surface my weaknesses
   - ❖ bruise my ego
   - ❖ take me down
   - ❖ make me face the truth / require me to step up

   and therefore I shut you down with:
   - ❖ impatience / believing that the problem is unsolvable
   - ❖ minimizing the concern / condescension
   - ❖ anger / rudeness / defensiveness / belittlement
   - ❖ arguing the "facts" / proving you wrong / over-simplifying
   - ❖ ignoring you / being obtuse / pretending it's not a problem
   - ❖ staying small / being too loud / panic / catastrophizing
   - ❖ enabling / nagging
   - ❖ tuning you out
   - ❖ body pain / illness

2) However, not listening creates repressed shame and blame that yields an energetic block in the body, often causing pain. What if I allowed myself to release both fear and pain and listen to your concern?

3) What if this act of active listening heals all? In the act of listening, we discover each other's unfulfilled needs. Once we uncover our needs, we remember that helping each fulfill our needs always creates balance in the universe. This balance leads to an abundance of solutions.

4) Because I now know that listening heals all, my new mantra is: it's a valid concern, let's talk about it.

It's Easier

Serenity Tuning Fork ⓔ/ⓔ

1) It's easier to be:
   - ❖ addicted
   - ❖ righteous
   - ❖ inauthentically confident
   - ❖ numb
   - ❖ angry
   - ❖ afraid / apprehensive / nervous / anxious / depressed
   - ❖ busy
   - ❖ sick
   - ❖ in pain / pessimistic
   - ❖ living in scarcity
   - ❖ restricted
   - ❖ making up stories in my head so I feel awful
   - ❖ stressed / hyperactive
   - ❖ fixing/trying to solve unresolved problems
   - ❖ doubtful/insecure/repel people and animals
   - ❖ dissatisfied/feeling cheated
   - ❖ scared

   than to feel my true emotional pain.

2) My true emotional pain is that loved-one did not think I was good enough which makes me feel useless and ashamed.

3) However, in truth, I use this shame to distract me from my genius because I'm truly afraid that my genius would separate me from the rest of the suffering humans that I know and love.

4) What if I work this chain backwards? I am now ready to fully embrace my genius because when I do, I discover that I am a perfect fit with the world and therefore I'm never alone. By accepting my genius, I never feel useless and ashamed and therefore I fearlessly explore my emotional pain. And then I no longer carry defenses against feeling my pain and my problems immediately resolve.

Sniff wild orange

It's Worth It

1) My _{dowse vertebrae(s) from image below} is weak because I'm afraid to stand in my power. This fear arises because _{loved-one} punished me when I spoke up for my needs, my gifts and my strength.

2) The spinal weakness is disrupting (white matter/grey matter) in _{dowse spinal nerve(s)/brain/spinal cord from image below} causing (pain/dysfunction/burning/weakness/numbness/tingling). Additionally, I unconsciously sabotage my strength with:
   - ❖ weight issues / health issues / financial issues
   - ❖ lack of success / stressful situations / jealousy
   - ❖ repressed voice leading to aggressiveness / disappointment

3) What if I embrace that challenges from loved-ones give me the opportunity to fully embrace who I am and what I know to be true? With this choice, my spine immediately strengthens while my issues resolve. I have now recognized that it's worth it to naturally and enthusiastically be me.

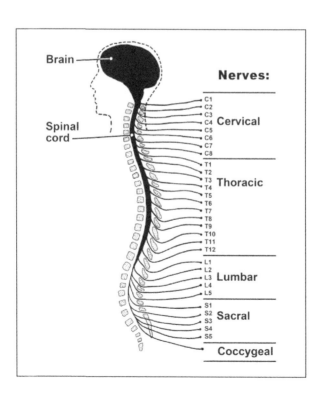

Just for Today

1) Because I see you as more:
   * popular / desirable / connected / social / cool / suave
   * easy going
   * productive / active / organized
   * successful / of a money maker
   * lucky / loved
   * brilliant / talented
   * doing "good"
   * creative
   * energetic
   * youthful / healthy

   than me, I try to make myself feel better with:
   * judging you / minimizing you / mimicking you
   * distance / hiding / absence
   * trying to fit in
   * raging against (my/your) flaws
   * lots of activity
   * numbing substances
   * trying to be the best / pressuring myself / overachieving
   * being your best friend
   * cleaning / organizing
   * cluelessness
   * getting attention

   however this usually results in a keen sense of failure actualizing as:
   * viruses/illnesses/heightened allergies
   * depression / anxiety / overwhelm / loneliness
   * exhaustion / sleep issues
   * obsession / hyperactivity / meanness
   * overthinking / the "shoulds"
   * stressful situations / headaches
   * paralysis

2) What if, just for today, I do my best to accept and love myself? And when I do, I simply no longer need to be like you in order to feel good about myself. Self-acceptance leads to self-actualization, which leads to joy, which leads to success.

Sniff wild orange

Leaping out of Bounds

Hold quartz crystal

1) I am afraid to leap out of bounds because:
   - ❖ I might get lost
   - ❖ I might love life too much – and what if I lost it
   - ❖ I might lose what I have
   - ❖ I might not be able to come back without damage
   - ❖ I might get into trouble
   - ❖ my tribe might find me unrecognizable
   - ❖ I might get labeled immoral or having a bad character
   - ❖ risk may lead to devastation
   - ❖ I might be unpopular or too popular
   - ❖ I might be too playful and others might be jealous
   - ❖ my power might bring substantial positive change which can lead to other's fear and criticism
   - ❖ it could create a roller coaster that's too hard to manage
   - ❖ I might be labeled irresponsible
   - ❖ I might fall flat on my face
   - ❖ I might get hurt (or you may think that I'm hurting you)
   - ❖ I might bring attention to myself with repercussions
   - ❖ I might get crucified
   - ❖ my loved ones might disapprove

   so I stop myself because it's too scary to leap and make a visible mistake which may present a depth of sadness that I believe that I cannot return from. Therefore, I am only willing to leap if the outcome is "above reproach."

2) What if I recognize that my heart is boundless beauty and that constraining my heart has kept me somewhat unhappy, unhealthy and ungenerous (mostly to me)?

3) What if I take the risk to create from my boundless loving heart? And what if taking the risk each day gets easier because I am compassionate to myself for anything that goes wrong? Then, I am no longer afraid, as I move forward, as I create a life that is beautiful beyond imagination, because my heart created it? And what if, one day, there is no experience of "out of bounds" because there is only love?

Serenity Tuning Fork

Lovable Being of Love and Light

1) I don't admire myself because:
   ❖ I am stuck in the **past** because _{loved-one} wasn't generous or protective of me and I'm waiting for that generosity to happen
   ❖ I am not enjoying the **present** because I'm not connected to my authentically healthy self because I tell myself that I'm not enough
   ❖ my desired **future** feels like a fantasy because I don't feel generous, cool or smart enough to be worthy of my special life

   I have felt that by not admiring myself, and therefore not standing out, I kept myself small and therefore, safe.

2) However, my lack of self-admiration leads to the lack of:
   ❖ good health
   ❖ loving relationships
   ❖ life affirming work
   ❖ financial freedom

3) What if I have it completely wrong? What if I'm supposed to admire myself because I am an extraordinary being of love and light? And what if once I admire myself, my gifts surface and my fantasy becomes reality? Self-judgment can no longer exist when I embrace that I am a lovable being of love and light.

Love, Acceptance, Health, Prosperity and Purpose

1) I cannot seem to tolerate the point of view of _{first thing that comes to} _{mind.} My lack of tolerance comes from the belief that this point of view is hurtful to me and my community and twists the facts. However, intolerance yields energy blocks actualizing as:
   - sickness / infectious disease / viral symptoms
   - memory blocks / body pain / exhaustion / nuisances
   - social anxiety / bleak anticipation / fear of imperfection
   - lack of: money / prospects / respect / community
   - hunger / weight / addictions / blame shifting
   - sleeplessness / restlessness / temper tantrums
   - impatience / obnoxiousness / demands / bullying
   - anxiety / depression / disordered eating / phobias
   - indecisiveness / lack of commitment / cluelessness
   - exhaustion / lack of direction / defensiveness
   - delusional / manufactured situations / resentment
   - over-sensitive / jumpy / overwhelm / insecurity
   - blame shifting / victimhood / lack of ownership
   - succumbing to a false narrative / false bravado
   - feeling inconsequential / feeling like I'm high maintenance

2) What if I can now allow myself to tolerate "intolerable" points of view through practicing compassionate inquiry? And what if I can do this because at the root all points of view is the universal desire to experience love, acceptance, health, prosperity and purpose?

3) I now choose to embody my divinely gifted vocation so that I can help others embody their divinely gifted love, acceptance, health, prosperity and purpose. When we embody our gifts, other's points of view no longer create defensiveness, instead it yields compassion.

4) I now understand that I am simply part of the whole. Within the whole, we each have unique gifts, talents and points of view. Our collective uniqueness gives the world its color and flavor. I no longer feel the need to fight you because that would be fighting me, because we are one and we make each other beautifully complete.

5) I have now infused my pain-body with a spiritual override and I'm now manifesting love, acceptance, health, prosperity and purpose.
Sniff lemon

Love Wins

Quartz crystal ☺/☺

1) I find myself worrying about the lack of reciprocation when I share my love with _{first thought that comes to mind,} which makes me feel flattened. This experience takes me out of self-love and sometimes I just want to dig a hole and hide in it.

2) But what if I recognize that my indomitable spirit cannot contain itself and crawls out of the hole as quickly as it went in because love can't stay hidden? And what if this act of crawling out strengthens my resolve and this time I'm less intimidated? Thus sharing my love gets easier? And what if when I resolve to remain loving no matter the response, then others lower their guard and open their hearts. And then I remember that love wins over fear.

3) I allow myself to remember that I AM divine spirit and I also remember that my mind and my heart create everything including enough self-love. This eternal memory helps me move forward without needing constant validation.

4) I now align my mind with my divine heart so that I can create heaven on earth. I AM creation and therefore I allow my loving world to manifest itself from within, so that I experience the magical and loving world of my creation.

Sniff wild orange

Magnificent Life

1) I have an unsatisfied urge to be completely loved for my _{first} thought that comes to mind. However, I can't get this urge fulfilled because my _{loved-one} primarily honored what they needed from me:
   - ❖ sweetness / to be a darling (less opinionated) / quiet
   - ❖ independence / tamping down desire / no demands
   - ❖ stillness / beauty / popularity / absence
   - ❖ thinness / submissiveness / conforming
   - ❖ athleticism / intellectualism / successful
   - ❖ maturity / responsible / self-sufficiency / stability

   because this made them feel safe. Therefore I feel shamed and threatened for needing what I need, so I react with aggressive expression. The feeling of rejection and the shame of my aggressive response can be so unbearable that I suppress the pain with conformity and the denial of my needs and my being.

2) Self-denial is an attractive tool because my mind compartmentalizes and avoids feeling pain and shame and helps me fit in. However, denial consumes a tremendous amount of energy and these energetic constructs block our natural flow, actualizing as a lack of:
   - ❖ success / money / freedom / acknowledgment
   - ❖ health / healthy relationships / true sexuality
   - ❖ happiness / self-assuredness / self-worth /
   - ❖ time / quality time with loved-ones

3) In the end, self-denial simply creates more pain, but embracing truth creates love.

4) What if I make the choice to choose self-love which means being myself even if I don't always fit in with my loved-ones? Once I give myself grace, I embrace my authentic magnificence and then others gravitate to me as I have so much love to give. When we all choose to be great and value each other's magnificence, together our stars shine bright and we create magnificent lives.

Magnificent World

Sniff lemon

1) My heart is unsettled because _{loved-one} did not give me:
    - ❖ love/kindness/veneration (deep respect)/consideration
    - ❖ honor/dignity/acceptance/inclusion/acknowledgement
    - ❖ the right to exist/a welcome into the tribe
    - ❖ attention/time/recognition/validation/understanding
    - ❖ freedom of: speech/voice/movement
    - ❖ intimacy/gentleness/healership
    - ❖ the benefit of the doubt/the time of day
    - ❖ support/conversation/companionship
    - ❖ room/privacy/truth
    - ❖ peace/calm/what I need to relax

    which makes me feel unworthy of goodness.

2) This love void is too painful to bear so I distract myself with:
    - ❖ illness/virus/infection/pain/allergies
    - ❖ stress/uncontrollable situations/fear of the unknown
    - ❖ lack of: money/success/fulfillment/health
    - ❖ sleeplessness/restlessness/boredom/being stuck
    - ❖ anger/disappointment/blame
    - ❖ addiction/worry/jealousy
    - ❖ lack of motivation
    - ❖ lack of: social-life/connections/belonging
    - ❖ self-loathing/shame/embarrassment
    - ❖ compulsions/obsessions/phobia/anxiety/depression

3) At this moment I choose to stop valuing my worth based on another's lack of kind attention because I now understand, at the deepest level, that their unkind attention comes from their feelings of lack of self-worth. I have now **broken the cycle** of pain and shame and I am free.

4) With this freedom comes my natural manifestation of love. In my realm of love, you can only feel love too. Therefore your love comes back to me in kind. WE ARE HEALED AND THE WORLD IS HEALED. We have now manifested a magnificent world.

Quartz crystal ☺/☺

Mission Complete

1) In order to achieve success, I believe I have to complete the seemingly impossible task of first thought that comes to mind. This situation is making me feel stressed and is creating:
   - ❖ headaches / congestion / cough / sore throat / fever
   - ❖ joint pain / body aches / body spasms
   - ❖ skin and hair conditions / allergies
   - ❖ poor diet / bad sleep / disordered eating
   - ❖ dreams feeling out of reach

2) What if in fact, I have unconsciously created this impossible task to distract me from fulfilling my loving mission of first thought that comes to mind? And what if completing my mission is my real fear because I am afraid that when my mission is fulfilled I will:
   - ❖ lack humility and no one will love me
   - ❖ be bored and my life would lack meaning
   - ❖ be threatening to others
   - ❖ feel like I need to stay on top
   - ❖ be unrecognizable in an unrecognizable world
   - ❖ be old / irrelevant / worthless / bored / unrelatable
   - ❖ leave this dimension / be dead
   - ❖ let people in and then get hurt (be vulnerable)

3) What if in fact when my mission is based in love (not about right vs. wrong), then accomplishing my mission is both grounding and ordained by the stars because when I succeed everyone will join me in my light? And if I recognize that if my mission is lacking love, I am easily able to alter course, because only love is natural and ordained. And what if now I am no longer afraid of my mission and therefore I don't block it in any way? And what if my stressors are now simply gone?

Quartz crystal ☾☉

Mutual Respect Creates Happiness

Serenity Tuning Fork

1) When we share spaces, and relationships, we prosper when there is mutual respect. But the human condition can often fall into disrespect.

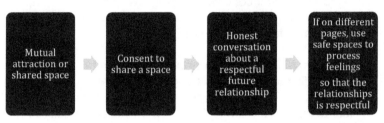

2) I felt disrespected when I shared a space or was in a relationship with first thought that comes to mind. I was never able to have a satisfying conversation about this and therefore it left me feeling drained, unlikable and lonely.

3) Without honest conversation, chronic viruses, addiction, and body pain develop to distract us from feeling the depths of the wound that disrespect surfaces.

4) The unprocessed emotion around getting disrespected is rage for the inhumane treatment received – this can lead to chronic body pain and/or fatigue. The unprocessed emotion for disrespecting others is guilt and shame which can lead to chronic congestion. Mutual disrespect leads to chronic coughs. *Breathe deep and see if you can get in touch with either when you were disrespected or disrespecting.*

5) Processing emotions around areas of disrespect clears guilt and blame on all sides and heals the wounds. This processing, leading to mutual respect, yields authentic connection and communication and happiness.

My Benevolent God-Power

1) Within this book's philosophy is the concept of *I create my own reality* and therefore I can create the reality of first thought that comes to mind. The concept is actualized by embracing my benevolent god-power described below.

I am love which means that I am the life force of all energy > Love is all powerful > Therefore, I am the benevolent god and can create anything that is love and extinguishes all pain

2) I have not allowed myself to embrace my benevolent god-power, which comes only from love, because I am afraid to be too powerful because I'm scared that:
   ❖ other's might distrust me or become jealous of me, then target and/or ostracize me
   ❖ institutions would fear displacement and try to hurt me
   ❖ instantaneous change causes too much disruption and life would become unfixable and unrecognizable
   ❖ using my exceptional power might create a catastrophe
   ❖ the loving, pain-free world would be unrecognizable and I would receive hate
   ❖ my power would deflate other's egos and power
   ❖ my success would create demand that I cannot handle
   ❖ my success would go to my head
   ❖ my loved-ones wouldn't get me
   ❖ other's suspicion of my power would cause me great pain and loss
   ❖ I would become judgmental of those that cannot ignite their love power
   ❖ I wouldn't fit into faith-based communities (because these communities are also pain-based)
   ❖ without challenges life would be boring
   ❖ to live without the thrill of conquering difficulties
   ❖ if it's so easy, we all can do it and then I'm not special
   ❖ my easy way would create a mockery of your hard way
   ❖ I would have too much power over you
   ❖ I would lose my creative inspiration because everything is good

3) What if I accept that my benevolent god-power is only fueled by love, and that **fear cannot exist in the space of pure love**? And without fear, our creations are only experienced and received as love? Therefore, with my benevolent god-power, I only create more love and all of our lives are forever changed to establish joy and peace for all. I can now choose, at this very moment, to create my enlightened reality of precious love and truly live happily ever after.

Sniff wild orange

My Bliss is Good for All

Serenity Tuning Fork

1) Because I create the reality of my desire:
   - ❖ pet's / family member's / friend's / my own
   - ❖ professional's / stranger's / famous person's
   - ❖ my body's / my mind's / sickness'
   - ❖ machine's / car's / technology's / object's
   - ❖ work's / studies'
   - ❖ politics' / lies'

   dysfunction is "helping me" actualize my desire for:
   - ❖ company / connection
   - ❖ success / happiness
   - ❖ enlightenment / healership
   - ❖ spirited movement / rest / stay home / relaxation
   - ❖ finding my: true self/truth/freedom/purpose
   - ❖ discovering my happy place / adventure

2) What if I recognize that I can create my desires without the aid of dysfunction simply by asking my heart to lead as blissful manifestation results? This simple act of heart-felt manifestation and joy has been blocked due to my fear of
   - ❖ criticism for my (selfishness/greed/laziness/lack of proof)
   - ❖ guilt if I'm not constantly producing something
   - ❖ guilt because it's easy for me when so many are struggling
   - ❖ having nothing fulfilling to do if I'm not fixing problems
   - ❖ lack of connection due to lack of joint problem solving

3) I'm ready now to release these fears and guilt because when actualize my bliss with ease, I can than easily show others the way.

Sniff wild orange

My Bright Shiny Star

1) What if in fact everything but love is an illusion? I am experiencing <small>first problem that comes to mind</small> from which I experience tremendous hardship. However, what if every hardship is simply here to direct me to love my enthusiastic self? Therefore this hardship is helping me choose to enthusiastically love my authentic (grace/joy/stillness/love/peace/fun/relaxation/health/wisdom/sexuality).

2) However, I have been afraid to love life enthusiastically because I was shamed for having too much (grace/joy/stillness/love/peace/fun/relaxation/health/wisdom/sexuality) by <small>loved-one</small>. Therefore I have blocked my authentically spirited self with:
   ❖ weight / allergies
   ❖ body pain / illness / body dysfunction / viruses / infections
   ❖ digestive issues / sinus issues / vertigo / headaches
   ❖ sexual dysfunction / untamed urges / tortured
   ❖ analysis paralysis / overwhelmed / sensory overload
   ❖ needy charges / feeling excluded / feeling dominated
   ❖ money issues / unfulfilled work / failure to thrive
   ❖ feeling oppressed / unkind relationships / gas-lighting
   ❖ skin issues / hair issues / teeth issues / breathing issues
   ❖ hormonal imbalances / depression / learned helplessness
   ❖ narcissism / low self-awareness / harsh narrative
   ❖ destructiveness / abuse
   ❖ denial / being clueless / defensiveness / can't read social clues
   ❖ accidents
   ❖ lack / financial issues / debt

3) What if standing up to projected shame and choosing to enthusiastically love life is always worth it, because now I discover joy, kindness intimate connection, and love? And what if when I embody my bright shiny star, you do too and together we heal the world.

Quartz crystal 〰◎

My Love Being

Sniff wild orange

1) I would like to shift into my love-being through releasing first thought that comes to mind, but I haven't yet.

2) My fear is that when I'm in a state of pain-free relaxation, I would no longer need my tribe, so I hold onto my tribe through the following defense(s):

Needed by Tribe	Not Outshining Tribe
❖ I see tribe-mates as less than so I can better and valued	❖ I have an internal dialog of why I'm not good enough which holds back my success
❖ I have skills! I have strength!	❖ I am embarrassed if I make a mistake which keeps me small
❖ I'm indispensable	❖ I follow your rules and definition of right vs wrong
❖ I'm a good follower	❖ I limit my world by breaking ties outside of my tribe
❖	❖ I experience lack and sickness so I am dependent

3) What if when I step into my love being, existing in a state that is unconditionally compassionate to myself and others, then the other members of my tribe feel so much love from me that my presence is always desired? Then the magic happens because when they feel my love, they choose love over pain as well. Now we are happy, healthy and successful.

Quartz crystal ☉⁄☉

My Loving Truth

1) I am experiencing a block in my _{dowse 1-3th chakra below,} because I am not projecting my truth. My truth threatened _{loved-one} because she/he/they were afraid of the consequences of projecting personal truth that may challenge community norms.

Chakras	
0 - Compassion (for my decisions)	7 - Remembering God-self
1 - Grounded/Secure	8 - Clearing Karmic Residue/Freedom
2 - Sexuality/Creativity	9 - Forgiveness leading to Optimism
3 - Personal Power	10 - Synchronistic Ease
4 - Love/Intimacy	11 - Instantaneous Transformation
5 - Joyful expression of Truth	12 - Ascending into Radiant Pure Joy
6 - Intuition/Honesty	13 – Unconditional Love

2) My truth block is actualizing as:
   * viruses / chronic fatigue / cough / infection / allergies
   * hunger / weight issues / blood sugar imbalances
   * lack of joy / lack of success
   * difficult charges
   * competitiveness / fighting
   * social-life interactions
   * freedom / disappointment
   * lack of kindness
   * insecurity / dependency

3) What if I remember that life can be spectacular if I embrace my truth at every juncture? Thus, as long as I speak my loving truth, even if it can be disruptive, then I'm liberated from fear. My loving truth that I'm afraid to share is _{state first thought that comes to mind.}

4) I have now regained my will to speak my loving truth (even if there are consequences). Now my life simply gets better, because I am authentically aligned to my heart. Inhabiting my loving truth always attracts more imitate connections, rather than loneliness. And so I choose to tap into and express my authenticity with grace and love.

Serenity Tuning Fork

My Gifts Heal the World

Sniff wild orange

1) I know that in truth I am ready to release _{first thought that comes to mind,} but I can't because I can't get over my anger about another's unloving point of view. *(Define point of view.)* My anger keeps me in unresolved _{choose grief state(s) below based on what resonates..}

2) What if when my loving vibration is lifted by using my gifts, the vibration of my loved ones rises as well? When my circle lovingly uses their gifts, this small circle creates circles of love and our collective vibration transmutes to love. This allows for the communal processing of grief, which resolves the anger. Unloving points of view retreat and the world is healed.

STAGES OF GRIEF

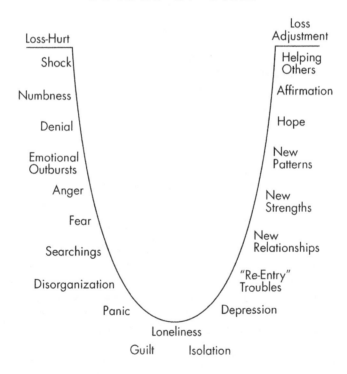

74

My Pet Makes Me Happy

Sniff lemon

1) Although I ask _{pet} to: *(choose as many as apply)*
   - ❖ behave/listen to commands/pay attention
   - ❖ follow the lead/walk nicely/understand limits
   - ❖ be gentle/friendly/polite/quiet/to not exist
   - ❖ treat animals, humans and the house with respect
   - ❖ be healthy/be quiet

   I recognize that this desired behavior scares me because I felt destroyed when I acquiesced with same behavior to:
   - ❖ loved one/parent/partner/children/friend/lover
   - ❖ employer/mentor/the "man"/colleague/authority
   - ❖ religion/community/God/traditional values
   - ❖ accepted practices/rules/expectations/norms
   - ❖ men/women/stranger/acquaintance/sexual partner
   - ❖ the universe

   and therefore, my pet's unwanted behavior is simply a reflection of my fear of being dominated by other's ideals, opinions and requests.

2) I now allow myself to separate from my fears because I give myself permission to create my life from my heart 100% of the time. I now recognize that following my heart's lead will always yield bliss and I therefore I never feel that I must acquiesce to a destructive paradigm. Now I am no longer afraid and I allow my pet to be easy, healthy and respectful.

Serenity Tuning Fork

My Vibrant Future is Today

Serenity Tuning Fork

1) I feel that my bold expression of:
   * joy / laughter / gratefulness
   * lovingly helping others
   * sleep / healthy foods / cooking
   * outdoor pursuits / sports / exercise / nature
   * learning / teaching
   * building / creating / the arts
   * romance / sexuality
   * rejuvenating projects / healership
   * satisfying work
   * socializing / conversation / feelings
   * vacations

   was not supported by first thought that come to mind. This lack of support has created the belief that my joyful expression is not valuable which yields embarrassment.

2) Embarrassment is an emotion that feels so uncomfortable that I tend to avoid bold expression with:
   * pain / sickness / weight / chronic problems
   * lack / limitations
   * isolation / boredom
   * rage / stress / anxiety / depression / panic
   * accidents / messes / exhaustion
   * allergies
   * alarming: behavior / problems
   * failure in: communication / electronics / protocols / digestion / growth / thriving / heal / consequences / mood balance / learning

3) What if I am willing to release embarrassment because I am no longer willing to yield my definition of value to other's judgment? When I boldly engage in what I love, my value naturally creates a life that supports me because everyone is attracted to my authenticity. Therefore I am always supported and loved.

4) I can now easily manifest my vibrant future because I am authentically and boldly me.

Sniff wild orange

On Top of the World

1) I'm totally anxious about separating from my unhealthy or unhappy relationship with _{first thought that comes to mind}, because separation might create (insecurity/unhappiness/loneliness/too much responsibility). In truth however, if I stay in unhealthy situations I create (insecurity/unhappiness/loneliness/too much responsibility). Additionally, leaving a situation that isn't working opens the quantum field of unlimited possibilities.

2) I can open the quantum field of unlimited possibilities with three ingredients: guts, authenticity and love. However, I have blockages in these areas as follows:
   ❖ **guts:** I'm afraid to have guts, because I don't feel protected when I take risks
   ❖ **authenticity:** I'm afraid to be authentic because loved-one refused to honor my true being because it conflicted with their choices for themselves.
   ❖ **love:** I'm afraid to love my choices because loved-one never achieved their dreams and I don't want to make them jealous or insecure.

3) What if at this very moment, I choose to jump because staying in place is creating unhealthy stress. Additionally, somewhere inside of me I know that jumping creates security, community, abundance, connected intimacy and happiness? And what if my courage inspires others to do the same? And now we're all on top of the world?

Quartz crystal ☉☉

Non-Judgment Heals the World

1) My parent(s) never liked it when I first thought that comes to mind. My fear is that if I don't control my thoughts, opinions and behavior, I will be judged by my (mother/father/both). Now I'm on edge and I don't feel worthy of my parent's love leading to a state of distrust of my parents, others, the world and me. This distrust and insecurity blocks the manifestation of my:
   * good health
   * loving relationships
   * life-affirming work
   * freedom
   * healthy desires
   * magic
   * glory
   * success
   * abundance
   * joy
   * movement

2) What if all the love that I need is inside of me? And what if this internal love is so pure that nothing can squash it? And what if all that I need to access this love is the acknowledgement that it's there? And what if at this moment of absolute enlightenment, I see myself as divinely perfect and I can no longer conjure up shame and distrust for my thoughts and behavior.

3) Instead I see the wounded pain in my parent's eyes and in my heart and with this recognition I am unable to pass judgment on myself, my children and all of humankind because I AM divine love. And what if at this very moment, my fear is gone, I'm healed and the world is healed?

Quartz crystal ☾◎

Peace, Love & Understanding

1) I find myself stuck in righteous conversation regarding:
   ❖ human rights
   ❖ lack of generosity / the top 1%
   ❖ religion / lifestyles / preferences
   ❖ other's choices, opinions and beliefs
   ❖ politics / mischaracterizations
   ❖ the universe's choices
   ❖ relationships
   ❖ hookup culture / purity / raw sexuality
   ❖ sexual preferences
   ❖ what a marriage should look like

2) What if this stuckness exists because I cannot give myself human rights because my right for physical, spiritual and financial wellness was criticized by _{loved-one}? Therefore I always seem to be on the defensive. And what if defensiveness is covering up a lack of self-care actualizing as:
   ❖ viruses / cough / congestion / Covid / Lyme Disease
   ❖ organ dysfunction
   ❖ chronic illness / chronic pain of feelings
   ❖ brain fog
   ❖ money issues
   ❖ power imbalances leading to disrespect
   ❖ misaligned: body/mind/spirit

3) What if I commit to practicing loving my needs because I now recognize that loving me, rather than shriveling based on past criticism, is the key to perfect health and compassionate understanding? I am now ready to energize the knowingness that self-care creates the space for peace, love and understanding which yields respectful interactions, yielding peace on earth.

Serenity Tuning Fork

Peace on Earth

Sniff wild orange

1) We can create peace on earth by releasing self-criticism.

2) Self-criticism arises because I was criticized by loved-one when I positively projected:
   ❖ genius
   ❖ fun / joy
   ❖ needs
   ❖ individuality
   Then I incorporated self-criticism as a means to keep myself in check with the aim of preventing other's criticism.
   However, this defense causes wounded pain and a lack of self-esteem.

3) In a state of self-criticism, our primary need is to be validated by others to make sure that we are okay and won't get into trouble. To ensure validation, I have joined a validating group with the same point of view: state first validating group that comes to mind.

4) In order to maintain our belief that our validating group is right, we need to find the enemy who is definitionally wrong. However, the need to always be right and make you wrong wreaks havoc actualizing personally as:
   ❖ viruses / infections / body pain / anxiety / depression / cough
   ❖ righteous politics
   ❖ social disconnection / bullying / a lack of nourishment
   ❖ insecurity / lack of success and forward movement
   ❖ grief leading to rage

5) Our collective problem is that the enemy "knows" that they are right and we are wrong. Then war rises up based on our need to continually claim our rightness.

6) If we simply accept self however, then the need for validation no longer exists. Then we have no need to prove our rightness and your wrongness.

7) When we work backwards, we discover that right vs. wrong is the illusion that we have created to deal with our wounded pain. By choosing self-acceptance, rather than needing to right, we create peace on earth.

Perfectly Energized

Hold quartz crystal

1) My light is lost in punishing exhaustion because I am afraid of:
   ❖ fun
   ❖ feeling rested
   ❖ being available
   ❖ optimism
   ❖ using my gifts
   ❖ health and happiness
   ❖ changes
   because this aspect(s) connects me to my true shining self.

2) I am afraid of my true self because I am afraid that my sparkle would cause others to shatter because of my misperception that:
   ❖ we can't all sparkle
   ❖ I would make waves that disrupt others
   ❖ my enlightened decisions cause disruption
   ❖ if I sparkle, I will lose touch with unhappy loved ones
   ❖ our distance would be painful and lonely
   ❖ it will cause others to feel powerless
   ❖ we won't need each other
   ❖ it would be too easy and therefore hard work loses its purpose
   ❖ others think I'm judging them and holding them to a really high standard
   ❖ we won't be rising above pain so we'll have no substance
   ❖ others will feel outshined, inadequate, whiney and angry and thus abandon me

3) What if I overcome my fear of reactions to my enlightened state, because I know that when I sparkle, others will join me in my light? When I'm authentic, everyone that I know (including me) knows that I will not judge them and therefore they gladly root for me and join me.

4) Now that I have embraced my authenticity, I naturally actualize my desires that emanate from my heart. My fear that my enlightened state yields harm, loneliness and a lack of purpose is replaced by love. And in a state of love all is fulfilling and beautiful.

Radical Self-acceptance

1) Because I don't feel worthy of:
   - ❖ loving relationships
   - ❖ happy family life
   - ❖ good health
   - ❖ abundance
   - ❖ life affirming work / getting hired
   - ❖ being attractive
   - ❖ a rich social life
   - ❖ fulfilling sex life
   - ❖ romance
   - ❖ care
   - ❖ rest
   - ❖ completed projects / tying up the loose ends

   I haven't received satisfaction in this area.

2) However, in truth there is control in feelings of unworthiness leading to a lack of manifestation. When there is lack, I'm doing the reaching for more and therefore since I'm the reacher, I'm doing it on my terms. If I were the worthy and popular one, people might be chasing me and that would feel like a burden. In this round-about way, I'm in control of the "yes". However, there is a void in the controlled "yes" because it leads to unfulfilled loneliness. My secret is that I have created a limited life because I'm afraid that I would lose control of my life if it were too busy, connected and expansive.

3) The healing for this is simple--it's radical self-acceptance. In this state we confidently express our truth which includes easily expressing tastes and limits. When we accept self, we accept worthiness and allow ourselves to be visible. Then our ability to manifest exactly what we want, at the right levels, actualizes into a fulfilling, connected and joyful experience. And then our mantra becomes: "of course it's going to be great, and so it is."

Serenity Tuning Fork

Relaxed and Happy

1) I want to freely relax, but I'm afraid to because:
   * I might get blamed for not trying or caring
   * I might become irrelevant
   * my flaws would be noticeable / I might say something stupid
   * I would do stupid things
   * I might not get what I want
   * I would be bored and fill myself with unhealthy and empty choices
   * I would be unimpressive
   * my people would think that I'm lazy and detached
   * the "shoulds" would fill my head
   * my worst self would show up
   * I would sleep all day / I wouldn't complete tasks on time
   * my freak flag would fly
   * I would be unrelatable
   * I might get hurt
   * I wouldn't take care of my people

2) Therefore, I keep myself unrelaxed by unconsciously creating a fearful state which squashes success and fulfillment. My biggest fear is first thought that comes to mind.

3) However, squashing relaxation with fear creates an energetic block actualizing as:
   * allergy/virus/sickness
   * feeling like a loser / social failure
   * the inability to move forward (analysis paralysis)
   * unhappy relationships / creepy behavior
   * stressful situations (financial/family/pet/work/friend/relationship)
   * pain / injuries
   * shame / drama / disappointments
   * exhaustion / memory issues / sensory blockages
   * the suppression of my gifts
   * OCD / anxiety / depression

4) What if freely expressing who I am and what I desire leads to success, fulfillment and relaxation? And what if squashing success, fulfillment and relaxation leads to a hellish existence. Therefore, there is nothing to lose by choosing to relax into my authenticity. When I do, I create abundant love and connection, while others join me in my light. I am now relaxed, happy and life feels like heaven.

Quartz crystal

Self-acceptance Heals the World

Quartz crystal

1) I'm frustrated by humanity because humanity just isn't doing enough to heal itself. This lack of goodness is blocking me from relaxing because I can't find a safe space in this crazy world.

2) Because the world is stubbornly unhealthy, I perceive that I must heal the world to find peace and relaxation. The weight of needing to heal the world is causing a block in my:
   ❖ lungs
   ❖ liver
   ❖ gall bladder
   ❖ spleen
   ❖ intestines
   ❖ bladder
   ❖ kidney
   ❖ heart
   ❖ muscles / soft tissue / bone
   ❖ subtle energy system

   because at times, I feel totally angry, useless and sad. But what if I stop waiting on the world to change because waiting is creating a pain body that is making me sick?

3) What if instead, I jump into the field of self-acceptance and within self-acceptance my gifts flourish? And what if humanity jumps into the field of self-acceptance because they can feel my accepting energy (because we are one) which feels so attractive because it feels so peaceful?

4) Our gifts fit together like a perfect puzzle. When using our gifts we intimately connect in a beautiful way, and through our kindness we each heal a little bit of the world. And voila, all the little bits create a healed and fully connected world.

5) And just like that I understand that self-acceptance is the key to world peace? And now I know that the answer is so much easier than I once believed.

Self-affection

1) Life seems to take a toll, while getting older presents itself as a multitude of issues including first thought that comes to mind. But what if this winding road of life doesn't have to age us because every cell in the body is new because the body is continually regenerating itself? And what if the key to allowing only healthy cells to duplicate is to have complete affection for my healthy self?

2) My lack of affection for my healthy self is a result of life's traumas. Affection for myself makes me feel vulnerable and lets down my guard to potential pain and trauma. Therefore, I unconsciously use a lack of health in for the form of:
   ❖ body pain / illness
   ❖ relationship struggles
   ❖ unsatisfying work / lack of funds
   to block self-love and affection which puts me on high-alert so that I'm on-guard for potential pain and trauma.

3) What if I have it backwards and self-affection, is what protects me from a painful and torturous life? And what if when I recognize that healing what is most traumatizing through self-love and affection is the only way manifest perfect health?

4) And what if self-affection simply clicks in because I allow myself to remember that I truly am amazing? And now that I remember who I really am, self-affection is now oozing through me and my brain is now reminding my body to only duplicate healthy cells.

Sniff wild orange

Self-love Creates Transcendent Beauty

Hold quartz crystal

1) From my (mother/father/spouse/children/pets/loved-one) I did not receive enough:
   - ❖ attention / prioritization
   - ❖ stimulation / fun
   - ❖ love / care
   - ❖ affection / sexuality
   - ❖ authentic encouragement
   - ❖ compassion
   - ❖ presence
   - ❖ respect
   - ❖ awareness of who I am

2) Due to this void, I am very sensitive to a lack of respect from (parent/loved-one/friend/my body/community/clients/lover/ co-workers/professional/God/faith/boss/helpers/strangers/ universe/profession/mind/teacher/hard work/social life/ popularity/finances/partners).

3) I am therefore filling the void with dramatic:
   - ❖ anger and resentment
   - ❖ body pain / sickness / nervous system disorders
   - ❖ turmoil / hormonal imbalances
   - ❖ regret / lack of success / delays / boredom
   - ❖ addiction / hoarding / unhealthy eating / cravings
   - ❖ judgment / anxiety / fear / melt-downs
   - ❖ fights / conflict / competition
   - ❖ heaviness / depression / exhaustion
   - ❖ sneaking around / cheating
   - ❖ numbness / distortions / sleep / emotional dishonesty
   - ❖ abusive relationships / conflicts / fighting
   - ❖ constantly being on / busy busy busy

4) The healing is self-love. When we allow self-love, we become self-respecting. Therefore we no longer are the victim in this drama. When I am no longer the victim, the void is naturally filled by me to me. When my love fills the void, I manifest all that is good for me. This allows me to create a life of transcendent beauty, which heals my world.

Sniff lemon

Self-love Fills the Void

1) I crave having more money. But what I really crave is what I wish that money could buy me:
   ❖ excitement / adventure / travel / fun vacations
   ❖ help / relaxation / down time / more time / peace of mind / stability / security
   ❖ people choosing to spend time with me / adoration / entertainment / being valuable / visibility
   ❖ more time with loved-ones / people being drawn to me
   ❖ comfort / luxury / time / the finer things / anything I want / better climate
   ❖ a cure / solutions / a body that ages well
   ❖ respect / power / self-determination
   however in truth I'm mixed on whether or not I want these things because of the be careful what you wish for mentality.

2) In truth, what I'm hoping for is that money can buy the things that fill up my love-void. I feel the love-void because I'm yearning for:
   ❖ objectivity / mature relationships / partnership / romance / intimacy / sexuality / touch
   ❖ friendship / deep connection / community / comradery / soul-mates / fitting into the whole / more time with loved-ones
   ❖ non-judgment / mind, body and heart stimulation / transcendent experiences / company
   ❖ appreciation of my gifts / affection / meaning / passion / fulfillment / acknowledgement
   ❖ laughter / serenity / freedom / ease / joy / perfect body function / vitality / all is always well / eternity
   ❖ parental love / love of children / relationship love / other's acceptance / confidence / receptivity
   ❖ compassionate understanding / integrity
   which I did not receive from love-one.

3) But what if the love-void is easily filled up with self-love because in self-love my high vibrational loving energy attracts only love and joy? And what if I'm afraid of self-love attracting all this joy because then I wouldn't have time for me, because I believe that joy requires me to be with others and I fear that I can't take care of me if I need to pay attention to you? This ultimate human conundrum (fearing loneliness and fearing having too much to do at the same time) is actually a false conundrum because when love creates joy, everything falls into place. Self-love leading to joy is our divinity and within divinity everything is truly divine.

Self-forgiveness Heals All

Sniff wild orange

1) When I choose to be life-affirming through:
    - ❖ joy / laughter
    - ❖ lovingly helping others
    - ❖ sleep / healthy foods / cooking
    - ❖ outdoor pursuits / sports / exercise
    - ❖ learning / teaching
    - ❖ building / creating / the arts
    - ❖ romance / sexuality
    - ❖ rejuvenating projects
    - ❖ satisfying work
    - ❖ socializing
    - ❖ vacations

    I'm no longer clenched. In this relaxed state, shame can surface and once surfaced, shame has the chance to heal.

2) At this magic moment I have a choice. I can clench and repress again, or I can allow what I'm not proud of to surface. When I'm not clenched, the shame has a soft place to land and my heart is able to forgive. I allow the shame of first thought that comes to mind to surface.

3) I can forgive this shame because everything that I do that feels unforgivable comes from the very human desire to be consequential and fit in so that I can secure love.

4) Self-forgiveness leads to the healing of mind, body, spirit and soul because in my relaxed, unclenched state, my qi flows freely as my blocks naturally resolve.

5) I have now unlocked the mystical magical path to manifestation and therefore I can now manifest first thought that comes to mind.

Shazam

Quartz crystal ☺☺

1) The painful circumstance of _{first thought that comes to mind} exists as a motivator to help me prove my value. This problem helps me prove my value because:
   ❖ solving this problem adds creativity and productivity to my life
   ❖ it's so bad that you must acknowledge that I'm doing my best
   ❖ it forces me to work hard and hard work is always honored
   ❖ it forces me to understand other points of view which gives me enlightenment credits
   ❖ finding the answer creates a solution that is so valuable that it is good for all
   ❖ it's torturing me to make me aware that I'm worthy enough to seek help
   ❖ we stay bonded and we lean on each other because of our problems
   ❖ it helps me embrace my healership
   ❖ it creates disappointment which keeps me ambitious

2) What if I recognize that when I'm enthusiastically myself, then I experience that I'm a natural asset wherever I choose to be. This shift reminds me that I am worthy of peace, love, happiness and rest. And when I know that I'm worthy, I no longer need pain to prove my worth. And then, shazam, I no longer collect problems and I'm happy, laughing, healthy and alive.

Strength and Joy

1) I feel uneasy embodying my authentic strength and joy, because loved-one showed disdain toward this and I am afraid to upset my loved-one and potentially get ostracized. I have unconsciously blocked my energy with issues I just can't seem to heal such as:
   ❖ chronic: illness / viruses / pain
   ❖ money issues
   ❖ under-performance
   ❖ lack of connection
   so as to remain in my loved-one's favor.

2) What if enthusiastically standing in my strength and joy is actually so life affirming that I am willing to allow the following pattern play out:

   a) I do my best to embody my strength and joy
   b) My loved-one shows disdain.
   c) I manage to continue to exist in my strength and joy even though it's hard.
   d) My loved-one is uncomfortable around my new-found strength and starts to squirm and escalates disdain.
   e) I watch the escalation, see my loved-one's fear with sadness, while recognizing their wounded shame and I discover my compassion. Compassion creates truthful understanding and allows me to release my loved-one's hold over me and I feel empowered.
   f) Embodying my strength and joy feels empowering and I now see my loved-one's disdain as childlike.
   g) While I continue to stand in my power, my loved-one's only choice if they want a continued relationship is to meet me where I'm at.
   h) I am now celebrating my strength and joy because I embody all that makes me me.

Success is Free and Easy

1) I would feel more peaceful and joyful if I created first thought that comes to mind.

2) I unconsciously block my success because I perceive that:
   - ❖ success may cause others to be jealous of me.
   - ❖ success may cause me to abandon others because of my lack of (time/space/patience).
   - ❖ success feels like enlightenment which others may perceive as weird or arrogant.
   - ❖ success creates too much work.
   - ❖ success creates a problem-free world…and then what would I do (it's boring).
   - ❖ I would become spoiled and lose touch.
   - ❖ If I lost success, it would be completely deflating.
   - ❖ success may cause other's problems to feel unrelatable.
   - ❖ true success requires me to embrace my ideals and I'm afraid that others would reject my ideal of first thought that comes to mind.

3) What if I allow myself to remember that success creates greater connection to my own and everyone else's hearts, rather than abandonment? And what if this knowingness regenerates my mind, body, spirit and soul? And what if the voice in my head that says, "this might be too disruptive" or "this might be too hard" is replaced with the knowingness that "I've got this?" No I am no longer afraid to create success.

Quartz crystal ☺/☺

The Easier Path

1) I have tried to cultivate _{dowse chart below word(s)} over presence, compassion, authenticity, joy, health and truth, so I don't get judged.

service	admiration	popularity	touch	gifts
adventurous	followers	independence	positivity	competence
animals	productivity	thriftiness	politeness	put together
appearance	being cool	impulsiveness	proximity	companionship
common sense	being interesting	not making a fuss	being impressive	being on-stage
winning	flexibility	neediness	fitting in	responsible
studious	politeness	appropriateness	submissive	resilience
cleanliness	sport	obligation	point of view	sexuality
Intellect / wit	beauty	charm	goodness	god fearing
possessions	personal time	progress	fitness	control
prestige	passion	invisibility	acquiescence	obedience
purity	good grades	entertaining	pain	romance
quiet	carefulness	enterprising	genius	being tough
resentment	power	loyalty	safety	liveliness
talent	conversation	stimulation	hard work	rest and sleep
thriftiness	success	craftiness	good times	independence

2) Cultivated traits can be hard to maintain because:
   - they aren't authentic
   - they don't come naturally to me
   - I can't always be perfect
   - It's too exhausting
   - they don't represent truth
   - it blocks my inspired journey

   and therefore when my cultivation fails, even a little bit, it surfaces my deepest wound which is that I don't feel love for the authentically natural me.

3) What if personal growth leading to happiness comes from choosing presence, compassion, authenticity, health, joy and truth over cultivating another's love and approval? And what if when I make this choice, my self-respect comes naturally? Within self-respect, the fear of being expelled from the tribe simply releases because authenticity feels better than ensuring other's acceptance And what if authenticity creates an easy world of personal glory, that is so magnificent that I never choose to dampen my authenticity again?

The Enlightened Path

1) I have taken a path that dimmed my bright star in order to avoid love-one's (jealously/upset) when I was too:
   ❖ attractive
   ❖ self-assured / confidently presenting myself
   ❖ successful
   ❖ sexual
   ❖ motivated
   ❖ outgoing / connected / powerful
   ❖ smart
   ❖ lively / fun
   ❖ emotional / needy
   ❖ relaxed / reasonable
   ❖ non-deferential

   I dimmed myself down with shame, aided by (weight focus / addiction / easily coerced / in pain / sickness / being a minor player / being unassuming / lying / shrinking / keeping my thoughts to myself / anxiety / stress / depression / OCD / situations that are hard to manage) leaving me in a state of insecurity and feeling irrelevant.

2) This subconscious choice to shut down stays with me because I am afraid of triggering, then being punished, by loved-ones when I shine. This unhealed wound keeps me in the tortured state of:
   ❖ low self-esteem / denial / over-sensitivity
   ❖ grief / aggression / cockiness / bitterness / pushiness
   ❖ indecisiveness / a lack of forward movement
   ❖ putting myself last / exhaustion / busy busy busy
   ❖ everything takes too much work
   ❖ minimal options / lack of success
   ❖ caring too much about what others think

   and sometimes I don't know who I am.

3) What if I give myself the freedom to release the subtle training by loved ones to stay small? In fact, our inherent nature can always shine through. When I allow myself to shine bright, my world is bright. And when I shine, my path is brightly illuminated, therefore my enlightened destiny presents itself. I now realize that I feel so much more love around me when I shine, then when I stay small and therefore, I'm no longer afraid to be me. I now have charmed life.

   Quartz crystal

The End of Suffering

Sniff wild orange

1) I believe that my life would be better and I wouldn't suffer if I had more:
    - love / friends / love-ones / community / connection / support
    - erotic sex / romance / relaxed environment / good news
    - drive / success / talent / recognition / kindness / luck / attention
    - money / beautiful things / prestige / class / dream house
    - beauty / health / youthfulness / adventure / a better view
    - working technology / body function / time / importance
    - strength / agility / know-how / boundaries / validation/ease
    - fun / stimulation / joy / compassionate understanding

    However it's my belief in lack that is actually causing my suffering.

2) I am experiencing lack and suffering because if I released suffering, religion would tell me that I'm not worthy of God's love because abundance yields sin and suffering builds a worthy character. *All of humanity holds these "moral" belief systems even if one is not religious because we, as part of the collective, consciously or unconsciously fear that losing God's love leads to a soulless existence.*

3) What if I could release these belief systems and allow myself to know that love of self is God and that love of self leads to abundance? And what if abundance creates more love, leading to more glorious abundance? And what if creating more:
    - love / friends / love-ones / community / connection / support
    - sex / romance / relaxed environment / good news
    - drive / success / talent / recognition / kindness / luck / attention
    - money / beautiful things / prestige / class / dream house
    - beauty / health / youthfulness / adventure / a better view
    - working technology / working body / time / importance
    - strength / agility / know-how / boundaries / validation
    - fun / stimulation / joy / compassionate understanding

    always fulfills my soul when it's aligned with my heart?

4) I now choose to share my heart with the world and then the universe fulfills my heart's desires in return. It is this fulfillment that builds worthy character because when I am fulfilled, I find it easy to be completely generous to all.

The Evolution of Love

1) Sometimes I feel that the sun doesn't shine on me because of persistent problem of _{first thought that comes to mind} In fact I have unconsciously held onto my persistent problems because without problems:
   - ❖ I might outshine my loved-ones everyone fearing that I might make them look foolish
   - ❖ I would have time, energy and money and would feel alone because everyone else is exhausted
   - ❖ I would be a free spirit, without cares (including caring for the world around me), and I would feel disconnected
   - ❖ I would be scared of the pressure of maintaining perfection
   - ❖ I would have no excuse to focus on me
   - ❖ I would become complacent and not be motivated to help heal myself, my loved-ones and the world
   - ❖ I would lack compassion because it's so easy for me
   - ❖ I would be frustrated by other's fights that are so important to them but would be meaningless to me
   - ❖ I would be considered a freak if I defy the commonly accepted laws of existence
   - ❖ I would be intimidating

2) What if in truth everyone is waiting for me to shine my light with such intensity that everyone would be happy to shed their problems because they can see through my choice that a life without problems is loving, connected, generous and beautiful? And what if when I decide to become the first human to shed all my problems, I spark the human evolution of love? This choice leads to the rejuvenation of the heart, both physically and spiritually, which leads to physical and emotional healing for all.

Quartz crystal ☺/☺

The Kind and Giving Universe

Phobias are the fear of non-conscious energy that can't be reasoned with; therefore phobias can't easily be resolved.

1) I hold onto the phobia of:
   - ❖ bugs/germs/animals/snakes
   - ❖ heights/falling/flying
   - ❖ crowds/small spaces/commitments/being dominated
   - ❖ flexibility/giving in
   - ❖ illness/pain/uncontrollable body function/chewing/death
   - ❖ sleep/sickness
   - ❖ weather/astrologic forces/water
   - ❖ mistakes/failure/public speaking/exposure
   - ❖ medicine/injections
   - ❖ exertion/socializing/aloneness/darkness
   - ❖ the unknown/strangers/other cultures/politics/people
   - ❖ not being able control my thoughts/gratefulness
   - ❖ not getting my needs met
   - ❖ being misunderstood/letting things go
   - ❖ other's not taking responsibility

   The nature of this phobia "helps" me avoid connected success because I'm afraid that connected success inevitably leads to disconnection and/or failure. This loss of (fulfillment/friendship/enlightenment/romance/deep love/money) seems too painful to bear.

2) Holding a phobia in place carries a strong energy that yields blocks in my (mind/body/spirit/soul) actualizing as:
   - ❖ Illness/viruses/infections/allergies/weight/addictions
   - ❖ headaches/financial stress/worries
   - ❖ disconnection/addiction
   - ❖ social anxiety

3) What if instead of using my phobia to keep me disconnected so that I avoid loss, I choose to jump into (fulfillment/friendship/enlightenment/romance/deep love/money). When I make heart-based decisions through the twists and turns of a well-lived life, I will always find myself in deeper and deeper connectedness which leads to happiness, overcoming the fear of loss. Now my mind, body, spirit and soul are in communion with the kind and giving universe.

Serenity Tuning Fork

The Leap into Self-Love

1) My biggest super-power is self-love. My biggest obstacle is self-hate. Sometimes I choose self-hate because if I chose self-love, I would easily actualize all that I wish for. Then, I would expect me to be perfect. Then others might expect perfection and I believe that I would be shamed when I complained or expressed my physical and/or emotional pain.

2) The leap that we can't seem to take is that if we exist in self-love, then we would actualize a pain-free life. Self-love heals all is the essential premise of this book. This premise is big and hard to embrace, but it's actually fear that is stopping us from choosing self-love.

3) I'm afraid to take the leap because I would be changing the laws of human existence and it feels too big. I'm also afraid that I would be in this other worldly dimension all alone and loved-one would judge me for being superior through my enlightenment. So instead, I sit in self-hate and cannot manifest:
   - ❖ good health
   - ❖ loving relationships
   - ❖ life affirming work
   - ❖ financial freedom

4) What if I recognize that everyone wants me to be a super-hero, because my authentic being is a perfect fit for the world? My self-love can never alienate people, it just begets more love because that's what love does. Therefore everyone can't help but follow my example and step into this pain-free dimension of life which manifests as the experience of being a perfect fit in a pain-free world.

Serenity Tuning Fork

The Love Game

1) It is the human condition to value self and others based on numbers. In my case I value myself based on:
   * my weight/number of calories/body stats/hours of sleep
   * grades/rank/number of good deeds/number of compliments
   * minutes or miles of exercise/ size of my house
   * number of success stories
   * salary/money in the bank/the size of my budget
   * paying the least for the best/being able to buy the best
   * number of social engagements/number of friends
   * number of kids (and kid's numbers)
   * amount of attention/social media friends and likes
   * age in regards to health and success/blood pressure
   * number of clients/customers/people I've helped
   * number of expensive toys
   * hours that I work/amount that I produce
   * my pain quotient / the happiness quotient
   * my rules being followed

2) What if I value myself based on a number so that I am always confirming how disappointed I am in myself because the measures that I lose in often outweigh the measures that I win in. I now become obsessed with fixing the losses. Trying to win in the numbers game is attractive because for some reason we want to spend our time punishing ourselves by wasting time because it often leads to disappointment.

3) Therefore, my actions suggest that what I value the most is wasting time. In truth, I spend my time wasting time on numbers because it's easier than spending time in human connection because human connection can be so exhausting because it can be hurtful, competitive and creates emotional drain.

4) The answer is quite simple. When releasing self-judgment and replacing it with self-love, then human connection no longer triggers us and therefore our relationships with each other are no longer hurtful and draining. Being with and connecting to others is now joy.

5) When we get closer to self-love, we begin to rip off the band-aid and allow more human connection. We naturally discover that the more we love and accept self, the more authentic we are. We then gladly give up the absurd numbers game and replace it with the love game.

The Memory

Quartz crystal ⊘⊘

1) I'm deeply afraid of _{first thought that comes to mind}. This fear actualizes as:
   - ❖ headaches / congestion / constant hunger
   - ❖ cautiousness
   - ❖ difficult behavior / negative attention
   - ❖ being shut down / guilt / inner turmoil
   - ❖ disease / ulcers / chronic illness / chronic pain / nerve pain
   - ❖ demanding behavior / lies / rage
   - ❖ a dampened spirit / overwhelm / exhaustion
   - ❖ anxiety / depression / hyper-vigilant / fragile
   - ❖ lack of romance (in life) / FOMO
   - ❖ sexual issues / body function issues

2) This fear and the associated symptoms are distracting me from re-experiencing a memory. *Close your eyes and allow the memory to surface.*

3) This memory is so charged because I felt:
   - ❖ unsupported / unloved / that nobody cared
   - ❖ assaulted / flattened / useless
   - ❖ out of control / reckless / unsafe / tortured
   - ❖ shamed / embarrassed / alone / unwanted / insulted
   - ❖ fraudulent / inconsequential / out of place
   - ❖ like a failure / like the worst / a lack of comprehension
   - ❖ like a killjoy / selfish / impulsive
   - ❖ mean / like a cheat / like a thief / like a liar
   - ❖ like a blame shifter / judgmental / immature
   - ❖ disloyal / shitty / like a jerk / wrong
   - ❖ unpopular / like I didn't fit in
   - ❖ inadequate / a lack of comprehension
   - ❖ uncaring / irresponsible / like I broke commitments
   - ❖ impure / like I led you on
   - ❖ lazy / silly / absent minded
   - ❖ like I created a frenzy / like I'm a nuisance / undeserving

4) Fear and associated defenses release when I'm no longer repressing feelings that I did something terribly wrong. Simply surfacing these feeling sets me free and allows me to easily love myself and others. This freedom releases emotional blocks stored in the body that disrupt body fluidity, thereby regenerating mind, body, spirit and soul. I'm healthy and at peace.

The Perfect Fit

Quartz crystal

1) Sometimes I experience stress regarding my relationship with (loved-one/friend/pets/body/community/home/everything/work/God/ethics/professional/teacher/boss/work place/customer/stranger/acquaintances/the planet/rules/health/humanity/being/mind/myself/my thoughts) because I feel like this relationship doesn't:
   - ❖ trust me/have faith me/nurture me
   - ❖ protect me/take care of me/prioritize me
   - ❖ include me/need me/want me
   - ❖ love me/like me/appreciate me
   - ❖ value me/listen to me/believe me/validate me
   - ❖ respect me/honor me/see me/know me
   - ❖ serve me/fulfill me/function well for me
   - ❖ see me as one of you/see me as worthy
   - ❖ share raw emotions with me
   - ❖ respect that the only love is real
   - ❖ last forever

   but in fact, first and foremost, it is me who feels this way about me as a result of how my parents saw me.

2) What if I choose at this very moment to drop my insecurities and believe that I am exactly who I am and where I'm supposed to be? I can do this because I am always on my journey to love myself more deeply? And what if this change of perspective is worth it, because then I've changed my reality to one in which I am a perfect fit. Therefore, it's easy for me to love, and when I love, I always know that I am loved. As a result, my stress transmutes to love.

Serenity Tuning Fork

The Upside of Hope

Serenity Tuning Fork

1) I choose to have hope that I can heal <small>fill in with unsolved problem.</small> However, having hope can feel like a roller coaster due to the upsides and downsides of hope.

   The upside of hope:
   - lifts the vibration
   - reminds me that all things are possible
   - gives me the ability to visualize a beautiful future

   The downside of hope:
   - disappointment leading to anger, sorrow and lost faith, yielding a very low vibration

2) In truth, hope is truth. The realization of a happier and more fulfilled life is the basis of creation. Disappointment only arises because I have fear (often unconscious) of the creation of my dreams. In order to release disappointment:
   a. Visualize life without <small>same problem in #1.</small>
   b. Search in your mind's eye for the negatives that can come from life without this problem. *You might not be able to visualize the negative because our problems are illusions.*
   c. I allow myself to remember that manifestation that comes from the heart, is loving, compassionate, and is always for the highest good for all.
   d. I now exist in the vibration of hope, love, and positivity as I release my problems. I am now at peace and have repatterned my world.

Sniff lemon

The Magic of Easy Manifestation

Serenity Tuning Fork

1) For the following questions, fill in with the first concept that comes to mind:

    a) What I want to heal is_____.

    b) What I want is to create is_____.

    c) What I really want is_____.

    d) What I really, really want is a kind, loving, abundant and supportive world for all.

2) The answers to the questions above naturally manifest when I embrace my desire for a kind, loving, abundant and supportive world.

3) I have unconsciously made a choice **not** to manifest my true desire for a kind, loving, abundant and supportive world, because I believe that to manifest all of this, relaxation is the key. However, relaxation feels unsafe because relaxation made me vulnerable to criticism from first thing that comes to mind for being first thing that comes to mind.

4) I can release the sting of this criticism by going within and accepting what I was criticized for by recognizing that this quality is not definitional, it's simply something I need or do sometimes. It is self-acceptance that creates relaxed vulnerability because in self-acceptance there is no criticism that I am not aware of and have not already accepted in me.

5) Self-acceptance is the magic ingredient for easy manifestation.

Sniff lemon

The World of our Dreams

Serenity Tuning Fork

1) Although I feel like I'm open-minded, in truth I'm afraid of opinions that conflict with my beliefs. My fixed beliefs originate from my unavailable _{loved-one} who didn't consider my needs. Not getting my needs met makes me feel vulnerable and therefore my strong opinions serve me by reducing my fear of not getting my needs met.

2) However, I'm now acting from a fear construct rather than from my heart. This causes me to fill the need void with:
   ❖ domination / competition
   ❖ suppressing dialog / tuning out / avoidance
   ❖ disconnecting from loving relationships
   ❖ taking charge / micromanaging
   ❖ repressing memories
   ❖ hiding / emotional dishonesty
   ❖ voting or choosing from a place of fear
   ❖ stress and distractions
   ❖ health issues / get sick so I don't have to connect
   ❖ bonding over communal unhappiness and betrayal

3) When operating from fear, dialog is shutdown, which creates the perception that my needs win. However, the shutdown can lead to an energetic block forming as: illness / virus / infection / overwhelm / angry mobs / disasters / headaches / unfulfilled promises / exhaustion / disconnection / body pain / disappointment / lack of success / lack of fulfillment / not fulfilling my potential / avoidance

4) Although allowing dialog can make me feel unsafe, deep understanding of all viewpoints yields a thoughtful and compassionate world. The benefit of this new world is that everyone, including me, feels heard and valued. Therefore I'm no longer in need of focusing on the void from unavailable loved-ones.

5) I now experience the world as a perfect fit, so I fearlessly and naturally fulfill my needs and find my place. We have now created the world of our dreams.

Sniff wild orange

Vibrant Life

Sniff orange

1) I repress my bold expression of
   - ❖ adventure/artistry/celebration/leadership
   - ❖ inspirational living/romance/laughter/magic
   - ❖ optimism/passion/playtime/fun/affluence/health
   - ❖ clear thinking/productivity/my true vocation
   - ❖ authentic conversation/freedom/using my voice

   because I believe that my authentic bold expression might cause me to receive punishment from first thought that comes to mind.

2) Needing to repress what I enjoy the most can actualize as an addiction to:
   - ❖ food/substances/work/too much to do/sex
   - ❖ passivity/anxiety/fear/sadness/misery/sickness
   - ❖ phobia/pain/exhaustion/drama/lack of sleep
   - ❖ difficult situations/feeling like the victim/stress
   - ❖ fixing whatever I perceive is wrong
   - ❖ other's control/intensity/analysis paralysis
   - ❖ fear of what other's think/shutting down conversation

3) I believe that the repression of my bold expression helps me avoid punishment. But In fact, expressing my passionate truth yields the end of punishment. Once I am no longer afraid of punishment, the punisher loses his or her power and I am free to be me.

4) When I am free, health and vitality return and I naturally live s boldly exciting life.

Serenity Tuning Fork

Books By Rebecca Cohen

Mystical Manifestation – Learn Divine Magic, a manifestation tool that accelerates the fulfillment of your dreams.

Divine Grids: a Celebration of Crystal Healing – Included are 80 pre-formed crystal grid diagrams designed to help overcome specific lifelong struggles.

What My Dog is Teaching Me About Me: Dog Training the Easy Way – This book decodes how your dog's unwanted behavior is mirroring your deepest fears. This book will help you resolve those fears, thereby resolving the behavioral issues as well.

Only Love is Real: a Book of Inspirational Verse (art by Shiya Stone)

My Path to Joy (with Lisa Orlandi) – A series of **Path** protocols that provide insight to help you remove your blocks to joy.

Plant Medicine, An Integrative Approach to Essential Oil Use -- A simple approach, delivering focused information on how to provide healing for the mind, body and spirit using specific essential oils. (**Essential Oils Book** is an abridged version of **Plant Medicine**)

Sound Medicine, Planetary Sound Healing for the New Age – A guide to using tuning fork vibration to tune our body, mind and spirit to our divine vibration. In divine vibration we are healthy, happy, loving and following our path.

Crystal Medicine for the New Age – A guide to using the beauty of crystal energy to transmute unhealthy crystalized body and mind formations to the body's natural state of perfect health and unconditional love.

Food Love Medicine – A guide to using the spiritual properties of food to enrich our lives. Natural foods contain all the goodness we need to heal mind, body, spirit and soul.

Meditate with Your Angels – This book is both a guide book to accompany the **Embraced By Your Angels** card deck and a stand-alone book which leads you through a meditative practice with your angels.

The Gentle Force with Path to Heaven Grids and Seasonal Resets – This book contains inspirational verses, healing grids and essential oil formulas giving you the courage to make authentic change. Authentic change is the path to joy.

Card Decks – by Rebecca Cohen

The Path to Heal Card Decks
available only at www.thepathtoheal.com

The six miracle decks are: Peace, Blessings, Ease, Love, Self-esteem and Abundance. Each contains 44 healing cards with beautiful images and affirmations. (art by Shiya Stone)

The five specialty decks are:
- Embraced By Your Angels (biblical angels card deck)
- Divine Consciousness (enlightenment deck)
- What If? Deck and guide book (opens unlimited field of quantum possibilities)
- Divine Incarnation and the I Am Deck and guide book
- You are an Angel card deck and coloring book with Jessica de Waal

The two loving tarot cards and guide books are: Doggie Love Tarot, Mystical Kitten Tarot.

For Russell

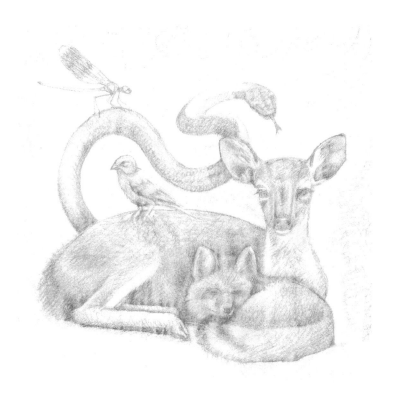

who facilitates my path to joy

Made in the USA
Columbia, SC
15 September 2024

41799120R00059